THE ARTISAN METHOD

THE ARTISAN METHOD

A Practical System to Stop Cravings, Quiet Hunger, and Restore Metabolic Health

Marco Bellini

Published by
Hearth & Vale Publishing

Published by Hearth & Vale Publishing
Imprint: Hearth & Vale — Practical Systems

ISBN: 978-1-7645239-1-2

This book is for informational purposes only and does not constitute medical, legal, or professional advice.

First Edition

Disclaimer

This book is for informational and educational purposes only. It is not intended as medical advice, diagnosis, or treatment. The author and publisher assume no responsibility for adverse effects resulting from the use of the information contained herein. Always consult a qualified healthcare professional before making changes to diet, fasting practices, or lifestyle, especially if you have a medical condition or take medication.

Preface

Most people assume their hunger, energy crashes, or weight gain mean something is wrong with them.

They are usually wrong.

The body is not failing.
It is responding — predictably — to food patterns it was never designed to handle.

If you are tired of fighting yourself, this book is not asking you to try harder. It exists because effort is rarely the missing ingredient. Most modern advice focuses on *what* to eat, or how much, while overlooking the factors that determine how the body reacts before calories or macros ever matter.

Those factors are timing, sequencing, and transition.

When food arrives too quickly, too often, or without clear resolution, the body compensates. Hunger escalates. Energy fluctuates. Weight becomes harder to regulate — not because of weakness or lack of discipline, but because the system is under constant correction.

This book was written for people who sense that dynamic, even if they have never had language for it.

Not because they lack knowledge.
Not because they lack willpower.
But because the prevailing models ignore how digestion, hormones, and appetite actually settle.

The Artisan Method is not a diet.
It is not a challenge.
It is not a belief system.

It is a practical framework for stabilising appetite, energy, and body weight by working with the body's mechanics instead of against them.

You will not be asked to count calories.
You will not be asked to track macros.
You will not be asked to live in restriction.

You will be asked to observe, test, and apply — to notice how the body responds when eating is paced, signals are allowed to complete, and absence is protected rather than feared.

This structure emerged through repeated real-world testing, not theory — by paying attention to what reduced effort rather than demanded more of it.

If you are looking for rules to follow, this book will frustrate you. If you are looking for clarity and calm, it will feel familiar very quickly.

Most people notice the change not on the scale at first, but in how quiet eating becomes.

That quiet is where everything else begins.

Table of Contents

How to Use This Book

This book is designed to be applied immediately.

You can read it straight through, but its real value comes from noticing what changes as you go.

Early chapters explain why hunger and energy crashes occur. Later chapters introduce simple ways to feel the difference directly.

The method works by stabilising transitions — between eating and not eating, between structure and social life — so progress does not unravel the moment real life intervenes.

You don't need to track anything to use this book.

Some readers, however, find it helpful to keep a journal and make a few simple observations at the beginning — not to optimise, but to *see* what changes.

If you choose to, you can note:
when you ate,
what arrived first,
and how hunger behaved afterward.

It doesn't need to be detailed unless you choose to.

Just enough to notice how order and pace affect how long a meal carries you, and how hunger changes when signals are allowed to complete.

This is not something to maintain.
It's something to use briefly until the pattern is clear.

Many people stop writing anything down once they realise they no longer need to negotiate with appetite. The body becomes the reference.

If at any point you feel unsteady, fatigued, or off-balance, pause and stabilise before continuing.

There is no benefit to pushing through discomfort here.

The goal is not control.
The goal is metabolic calm.

CHAPTER 1 — Why This Book Exists

Most eating problems persist not because of what we eat, but because digestion is never allowed to finish.

If you are reading this, there is a good chance you have already done everything you were told was supposed to work.

You've eaten less.
You've tried to be disciplined.
You've followed plans that promised certainty if you just stayed consistent.

And at some point, something always went wrong.

Maybe it was the evenings — where control seemed to disappear even though you had "been good" all day.
Maybe fasting felt possible once, then harder every time you tried again.
Maybe keto worked until it suddenly didn't, and when it failed, it failed completely.
Maybe the scale moved, then stopped, then reversed — even though nothing obvious had changed.

What hurt most wasn't the weight.

It was the confusion.

You didn't feel lazy or careless.
You felt like your body had stopped responding to effort.

That's a specific kind of exhaustion — the kind that comes from doing the right things and watching them stop working anyway.

Most people reach the same conclusion at that point. They assume the problem must be them — that they are missing some trait other people have. More discipline. Better consistency. Stronger willpower.

This book exists because that conclusion is wrong.

What you were experiencing was not a failure of character or commitment. It was a predictable physiological response to the way food now enters the body — too quickly, too often, and without enough structure for the system to regulate smoothly.

Most modern eating problems are not about how much you eat.

They are about **speed**, **sequence**, and **signal overload**.

When food arrives quickly, insulin rises sharply.
When insulin rises repeatedly, hunger escalates.
When hunger escalates, control eventually breaks — not because of weakness, but because the system is under constant correction.

Have you've ever felt like you were negotiating with your own appetite — delaying it, suppressing it, or trying to outlast it?

That wasn't imagined. You were responding to real signals generated by an unstable system.

This book does not ask you to fight those signals.

It shows you why they appear — and how they quiet when the conditions that provoke them are removed.

Nothing here depends on belief or motivation.

This book does not ask for agreement up front.
It is built around observation — what reliably happens when eating speed, sequence, and timing change under real conditions.

You don't need to believe the explanation for it to work. You only need to notice what changes when the conditions change.

Once the mechanics are clear, the relief comes first.
Change follows quietly.

The Real Problem: Instability

Most people who struggle with weight, cravings, or energy do not lack discipline.

They lack **stability**.

Hunger arrives unpredictably.
Energy drops without warning.
Cravings spike at exactly the wrong moment.

Food decisions accumulate until effort gives out — not suddenly, but gradually.

Over time, people adapt to this instability. They stop experimenting and start managing damage. They learn which hours are hardest. They plan around crashes. They snack. They tell themselves they just need to be more careful next time.

When this repeats long enough, the assumption becomes internal:

"This is just how I am around food."

It isn't.

The issue is that most eating systems — diets, plans, challenges, even many fasting protocols — are built around the wrong assumption. They treat appetite as something to control, suppress, or override.

So they rely on rules.

Eat this, not that.
Stop at this point.
Resist until the window closes.
Start again when it collapses.

As long as appetite remains quiet, these systems appear to work. When it doesn't, they fail — not because the person did, but because the structure never accounted for instability under real conditions like stress, fatigue, travel, or imperfect weeks.

This is why the same pattern repeats across wildly different approaches.

A plan works.
Hunger stays manageable for a while.
Then something shifts.

Meals stop holding.
Cravings arrive earlier.
Energy dips become harder to manage.
Mental effort increases.

At that point, people do what they've been taught to do: they tighten control.

Sometimes that restores order briefly.
Often it makes the instability worse.

Because the problem was never a lack of rules.

It was the absence of an underlying **rhythm**.

Why Structure Matters More Than Control

Human appetite evolved inside repeating patterns — not perfect ones, but structured ones. Periods of eating. Periods of rest. Variation across days. Natural pauses that allowed signals to settle before the next input arrived.

Modern eating removes those stabilisers.

Food is always available.
Meals blur into snacks.
Energy arrives quickly and repeatedly.
The system is never allowed to finish one job before starting the next.

In that environment, hunger stops being a clear signal and becomes constant noise.

People experience this as being "out of control," even when they are eating reasonably. Food occupies mental space not because it is desired, but because the system never fully settles.

Most modern methods never name this failure.

Public nutrition advice is designed to reduce harm across populations; this book focuses on resolving signals within an individual system.

They manage *what* you eat and *how much* you eat, while ignoring the structure that determines whether appetite becomes calm or chaotic in the first place.

The solution is not more discipline.

It is a structure that makes discipline largely unnecessary.

That structure is not about restriction.
It is about **rhythm** — how eating events are sequenced across a day and a week so hunger arrives on time, with the right intensity, and then quiets again.

Once that layer is addressed, many struggles people blame on themselves resolve without force.

The One Concept That Changes Everything

The simplest way to understand what's been missing is this:

It isn't calories.
It isn't willpower.
It isn't even food quality on its own.

It is **speed**.

Specifically, the speed at which food turns into usable energy in the bloodstream — and how the body is forced to respond when that speed is too high.

When energy arrives slowly, the system stays quiet.
When it arrives quickly, the system must correct.

Fast Input → Insulin Spike → Correction → Hunger Noise Slow Input → Signal Completion → Quiet → Stability

Those corrections are what you experience as crashes, cravings, and urgent hunger.

This is why some meals feel fine while you're eating them, then unravel an hour later. It's why certain foods seem impossible to stop once started, and why the desire for more often appears after you've already eaten enough.

Once you see this, confusion clears quickly.

You stop asking why hunger keeps returning.
You start noticing when it appears — and what preceded it.

Meals that hold release energy gradually.
Meals that collapse release it all at once, then force the body into cleanup mode.

That cleanup is not comfortable — and it isn't optional.

The body always prioritises balance over comfort.

If you reduce the speed that triggers those corrections, hunger changes character. It arrives later. It arrives softer. And when it passes, it actually passes.

This is not about eating less.

It's about allowing the system to finish one job before starting the next.

Everything in this method builds from that single principle though.

The exact timeline varies by person, history, stress, and prior dieting — but the direction of change is remarkably consistent.

When the Noise Went Quiet

I noticed it one afternoon without trying to.

There was no breakthrough moment. No discipline involved. I was partway through the day when something felt different — not better, just quieter.

Food hadn't crossed my mind for hours.

Not as a background negotiation.
Not as something to manage later.

It wasn't fullness.

It was completion.

The system had finished what it needed to do — and because it had, it stopped asking for input.

That moment reframed everything.

Not because it was dramatic, but because it was ordinary. I wasn't "being good." I wasn't following rules. I wasn't in a special state.

The system had simply been allowed to run at a speed it could handle.

Once you've felt that quiet, it's hard to ignore.

You start noticing how often hunger isn't hunger at all — it's correction in progress. A system responding to something that arrived too fast and left too abruptly.

The goal was never to eat less.

It was to stop creating situations the body has to clean up after.

What This Book Is Doing

This is not a diet. It is not a calorie-counting system.
It does not require food elimination.
It does not promise uniform outcomes.
It does not replace medical care.

There are no targets to memorise and no demand for perfect weeks. Nothing here requires pushing through hunger or proving discipline.

This book is about **structure**, not control.

Specifically, it introduces two layers that work together:

- **Meal pacing** — sequencing food within a meal so energy enters the system at a manageable speed.

- **Weekly rhythm** — arranging eating and resting days so signals have time to settle instead of stacking.

Neither layer works by forced restriction.
Both work by **timing**.

Nothing here asks you to fight your environment or isolate yourself socially. The system is designed to hold through imperfect weeks — because most weeks are.

If something doesn't reduce hunger, quiet cravings, or make eating feel less urgent, it doesn't earn a place.

This book isn't meant to be inspiring.

It's meant to be **useful.**

If you use it lightly, you'll still benefit.
If you use it fully, it should eventually stop needing your attention at all.

This book moves at the speed the system it describes needs in order to be seen clearly, without compressing itself for momentum or payoff.

That's the standard it's built to meet.

Why Rhythm Works in the Body (The Part No One Told You)

There is a part almost no one ever explains — the part that makes the next chapters necessary rather than optional:

Your hunger system has not been failing because of what you eat.
It has been misfiring because of *when* and *how often* food arrives.

Your metabolism isn't broken.
It's confused.

And that confusion shows up in specific, repeatable ways:

- hunger signals firing earlier each day,

- insulin rising too often and staying elevated,

- cravings driven by reward pathways that never fully shut off,

- energy arriving quickly and disappearing just as fast,

- the fuel switch between glucose and fat never completing,

- the body acting as if food scarcity and overload are happening at the same time.

This isn't a discipline problem.
It's a signalling problem.

In a stable system, hunger is not triggered by crisis or shortage. It tends to appear when the previous intake has been processed, insulin has settled, and the body is no longer correcting. In that state, hunger is a readiness signal — not an emergency.

When food arrives too quickly or too often, that completion never occurs. Hunger then appears early, loudly, and persistently, not because fuel is missing, but because signals are overlapping.

The moment timing becomes predictable — not perfect, just predictable — the body starts correcting itself:

- hunger waves shift later and soften,

- insulin patterns flatten,

- fat becomes a stable fuel instead of a backup system,

- cravings lose urgency,

- mental noise around food fades.

None of this requires effort.
It happens automatically once the environment stops forcing constant correction.

But the real shift — the one that makes this method compound instead of stall — comes from processes you don't feel directly:

- the point where insulin drops far enough for switching to begin,

- the point where cellular cleanup turns on,

- the point where digestion and appetite stop competing,

- the point where the body no longer treats hunger as an emergency.

You don't need to understand those mechanisms yet.
But once you do, the method will stop feeling like a strategy and start feeling inevitable.

Try A One-Meal Test of Food Pacing

You don't need to change what you eat to test the central idea of this book.
You only need to change **the order and timing**.

This is not a diet experiment.
It's a short observation that lets you feel how pacing alters hunger without restriction, belief, or effort.

Day One — Your Normal Pattern

For lunch, eat what you normally eat.

This can be fast food, takeaway, or a familiar meal you already know well.
Do not over-order and do not under-order. Eat the amount you

would usually choose without thinking about it.

When you finish eating, note the time.

Go about your day as you normally would.

When you first feel **genuinely hungry again** — not bored, not snack-curious, but hungry enough that food feels necessary — note the time.

At that moment, take a few seconds to notice how you feel:

- calm or restless
- steady or foggy
- neutral or irritable

There is no right answer. You are not judging anything. You are just observing.

Day Two — Change the Order Only

The next day, prepare or buy a simple salad.

It does not need to be elaborate.
Leafy greens, a vinegar-based or sugar-free acidic dressing, and a small amount of oil are enough.

When you are ready to eat lunch, note the time and eat the salad first.

When you finish, wait **ten minutes**.
Drink water if you like, but eat nothing else.

After the ten minutes, eat the same type of lunch you had the day before — the same category of food, prepared in the same way.

Again, eat normally. Do not restrict. Do not compensate.

When you later feel genuinely hungry, note the time.
Notice your emotional state using the same words you used the day before.

Compare the Two Days

You did not change calories.
You did not eat "clean."
You did not add discipline.

Only the **pacing** changed.

Most people notice at least one of the following:

- fullness lasts longer than expected

- hunger returns later

- hunger feels quieter rather than urgent

- the desire to keep eating fades sooner

- mood and focus remain steadier

If you didn't notice much the first time, repeat the test once or twice.
Patterns tend to become obvious with repetition.

This small difference is not willpower.
It is mechanics.

What you just felt is the effect of slowing the first wave — a preview of what rhythm does across an entire week.

You don't need to understand why yet.
That comes next.

This simple test shows how sequencing changes appetite immediately. If you want a clearer baseline after finishing the method, the Appendix on the Fast Meal vs Slow Meal test isolates the same effect by changing only digestive interruption, not food.

The next chapters explain what your body has been trying to do all along — and why giving it the right rhythm finally lets it succeed.

Who This Book Is For — and Who It Isn't

This book is written for people who are tired of managing food as a constant problem.

It is for those who have tried to eat less, eat better, eat cleaner, or eat more carefully — and found that effort alone never quite solved the instability underneath. It is for readers who want eating to take up less mental space, not more.

This book will likely resonate if:

- hunger feels unpredictable or intrusive,

- meals don't seem to "hold" the way they used to,

- fasting works sometimes but collapses under stress,

- or food decisions feel louder than they should.

It is especially suited to readers who are willing to observe patterns without forcing outcomes — and who are open to structure that works quietly rather than through control.

This book may not be a good fit if you are looking for:

- a meal plan,

- a food list to follow precisely,

- a calorie or macro target,

- or a short-term weight-loss protocol.

It is also not designed as a performance system or optimisation framework. If your goal is to push limits, chase metrics, or maximise outcomes aggressively, this approach may feel intentionally underpowered.

Nothing here requires perfection, compliance, or belief.
The method works by changing conditions — not by demanding effort.

How to Read the Rest

You don't need to read this book in order.

Some readers want the explanation first.
Others want proof.

Both approaches work.

Start by noticing outcomes, not rules.

Meals that hold longer.
Hunger that arrives later.
Days that feel quieter than expected.

If those improve, you're on the right track — even if you haven't read everything yet.

Next we show how the mechanics become concrete, and where most people begin seeing immediate feedback.

You don't need to agree with what's coming.

You just need to try it and notice what happens.

CHAPTER 2 — Why We Crash, Crave, and Gain Weight

The Pattern Most People Live Inside

Most people don't gain weight simply because they eat constantly.

They gain weight because their days follow a repeating sequence — one that never allows energy to fully settle before more is added.

Energy arrives quickly.
It drops just as quickly.
Something is used to patch the gap.
The cycle restarts.

Over time, this becomes the background rhythm of daily life.

You eat, and things feel fine for a while. Then focus fades. Hunger shows up earlier than expected — not a gentle hunger, but a distracting one. You reach for something small, something quick, or something that feels earned.

Relief is brief.
The drop returns.

By late afternoon or evening, decisions feel heavier. Portions drift. Cravings become more specific. Restraint feels unreasonable — not because you don't care, but because the system is already unstable.

This sequence is often interpreted psychologically.

People are told they're emotional eaters. Stress eaters. People who "lose control."

But the order matters.

The crash comes first.
The craving follows.
The snacks are an attempt to stabilise what already feels off.

In those moments, the body isn't asking for more food.

It's asking for **stability**.

When energy arrives in sharp bursts, the body has to correct aggressively. When those corrections overshoot, the signal that follows feels like hunger — even when total intake has been more than sufficient.

That response isn't a mistake.

It's the system doing its job inside an environment that keeps forcing it to correct.

Once this pattern repeats often enough, weight gain becomes easier — not because of indulgence, but because the system rarely finishes one cycle before the next begins.

This chapter slows that loop down.

Not by asking you to eat less.
Not by asking you to resist cravings.

But by showing you where instability actually starts.

When Food Moves Too Fast

The crash–crave cycle doesn't begin with overeating.

Modern food converts into usable energy far faster than the body evolved to manage comfortably. When that energy arrives slowly, it's absorbed, used, and cleared before the system asks for more.

When it arrives quickly, everything compresses.

Energy spikes.
The body corrects aggressively.
Levels fall faster than expected.

What isn't used or resolved doesn't disappear. It's set aside for later — cleared from circulation so the system can stay stable. The problem is that "later" often never arrives cleanly.

The signal that follows feels like hunger — but it's not a deficit. It's a response to a **drop**.

This is why people can eat a large meal and still feel compelled to snack soon after. It's also why certain foods seem impossible to stop once started. They don't fail to satisfy — they convert too fast to settle.

Texture matters.
Processing matters.
Combinations matter.

Soft, refined foods break down quickly.
They move through digestion faster than the body evolved to manage comfortably.

The body receives a surge it didn't request — then has to clean it up.

That cleanup is what creates the crash.

Once the crash begins, appetite becomes reactive. Eating decisions gain urgency. Portions drift not because of indulgence, but because the system is trying to prevent another drop.

Calories don't explain this.

Two meals with the same energy content can behave completely differently depending on how fast that energy enters circulation.

One holds.
The other collapses.

And the difference isn't discipline.

It's conversion speed.

Why This Pattern Is Everywhere Now

Once speed is understood, the pattern stops looking personal.

It looks environmental.

Most people aren't eating unusually large amounts of food.
They're eating food designed — deliberately or incidentally — to move through the body as efficiently as possible.

Refining removes structure.
Grinding increases surface area.
Cooking softens fibres.
Combining starch with fat accelerates absorption further.

None of this is malicious. It makes food cheap, palatable, and easy to consume.

It also means energy arrives faster than the body can comfortably regulate.

That's why the same cycle appears across lifestyles and cultures. It shows up in people who eat "clean," people who cook at home, and people who are actively trying to do the right thing.

The pattern doesn't require excess.

It only requires repetition.

Fast meals during the day.
Energy swings in the afternoon.
Overcompensation at night.

Even weekends rarely reset it. They often intensify it.

This is why advice focused on restraint struggles to hold. It asks people to swim against a current they don't realise is there.

It also explains why many people feel worse when they try to eat better. They remove obvious indulgences but keep the same speed. Meals still collapse. Hunger still escalates. Effort increases without relief.

That's not a failure of commitment.

It's a mismatch between the advice and the environment it's being applied in.

Once this clicks, the question changes.

You stop asking why you can't stick to a plan.

You start asking why the plan never accounted for speed at all.

The Moment Meals Tip From Stable to Chaotic

Not all meals behave the same way.

Some leave you steady for hours.
Others unravel quickly — even when the portions look
reasonable.

The difference shows up at the **beginning** of the meal.

When the first thing the body receives converts quickly,
digestion accelerates immediately. Signals stack early.
Corrections begin before the meal is finished.

By the time eating stops, the system is already shifting into
cleanup signalling.

That's when stability is lost.

Meals that start slowly behave differently.

When the first inputs take time to break down, digestion sets a
measured pace. Energy enters circulation gradually. The rest of
the meal is absorbed into that slower rhythm.

Nothing spikes.
Nothing needs urgent correction.
Hunger arrives later — and softer.

This is why meals that look similar on paper can feel completely
different in practice. It's not randomness. It's **sequence**.

Once the opening of a meal sets the speed, everything

downstream follows.

Trying to fix a meal after it has already accelerated rarely works. Adding more food doesn't restore stability — it often deepens the crash.

The simplest way to change the outcome is to change the beginning.

The Small Shift That Changes the Whole Day

At this point, the pattern should be clear.

Fast energy first leads to early correction.
Early correction leads to urgent hunger.
Urgent hunger drives reactive eating later in the day.

The shift that interrupts this loop is small.

You don't need to overhaul meals.
You don't need to track intake.
You don't need to remove foods you enjoy.

You only need to change **what arrives first**.

When a meal begins with slower inputs, digestion sets a pace the body can manage. Energy spreads out. Corrections soften.
Hunger becomes predictable instead of urgent.

Most people have experienced this without recognising it.

A lunch that held unexpectedly.
An afternoon that stayed steady.
An evening without the usual pull toward snacking.

Those aren't coincidences.

They're signs the meal started at a speed the system could handle.

This is the first place where the method proves itself.

Try it once and you'll feel the difference before you reach for anything else.

Not dramatically.
Quietly.

A longer gap before hunger returns.
A steadier afternoon.
Less urgency around food.

That feedback matters more than explanation.

Because once you feel it, the rest of the system stops sounding theoretical.

In the next chapter, we'll turn this into something deliberate — laying out the simple sequencing pattern that stabilises meals without restriction or complexity.

You won't be asked to memorise rules.

You'll be asked to notice what works — and repeat it.

CHAPTER 3 — How to Eat Without Triggering Crashes

Why Order Matters More Than Choice

By now, a pattern should be emerging.

The difference between a meal that holds and one that collapses usually has less to do with *what* you ate than *how the meal unfolded.*

This runs against most advice.

People are trained to think in terms of ingredients — good foods, bad foods, better swaps. Choice becomes the focus.

But the body doesn't experience meals as lists.

It experiences them as **sequences**.

What arrives first sets the pace.
What follows is processed inside that pace.
And once the speed is set, the rest of the meal tends to follow it.

This is why two meals containing the same foods can produce very different days.

When fast-converting foods arrive early, digestion accelerates immediately, and what follows enters a faster-moving system. Energy enters circulation quickly. Corrections begin sooner. Hunger returns earlier — often with urgency.

When slower inputs arrive first, digestion establishes a measured rhythm. Energy spreads out. Signals stay orderly. The rest of the meal is absorbed without disruption.

Nothing mysterious is happening.

The system is responding to order.

That distinction matters.

If instability were caused by "bad foods," the solution would be avoidance.
If it were caused by excess, the solution would be restriction.

But if instability is caused by **sequence**, the solution is neither.

It's pacing.

Once you see this, pressure drops. You don't need perfect meals or rigid rules. You only need to notice which foods set the speed — and which ones allow the system to settle first.

The leverage point is early.

That's where small changes produce the largest effect.

How Different Foods Set the Pace

Not all foods move through the body the same way.

Some take time to break down.
Others convert quickly.
Some accelerate whatever pace is already in motion.

Foods with intact structure — things that require chewing and digestion — tend to slow energy release. They occupy the system long enough for signals to remain steady.

Refined or soft foods tend to do the opposite. They break down rapidly. Energy arrives early. The body has less time to regulate the flow.

Protein sits between these extremes.

It doesn't convert into energy quickly, but it does stimulate digestion. When protein enters a fast-moving environment, it can accelerate the process. When it enters a slower one, it settles into that pace.

This is why the same food can feel stabilising in one context and destabilising in another.

A food is rarely the problem in isolation.
It becomes a problem **by when it arrives**.

Meals that begin with fast-moving inputs often set a pace the rest of the meal cannot slow down. Meals that begin with slower inputs tend to absorb faster foods later without issue.

You can think of the sequence this way: **structure first, fuel last** — not as a rule, but as a description of what allows digestion to settle before energy ramps up.

Most people have felt this difference without naming it.

A lunch that unexpectedly holds for hours.
Another that unravels quickly despite similar portions.
Same foods. Different order. Different outcome.

Digestion isn't just about breaking food down.

It's about managing **flow**.

Once that clicks, the rest becomes predictable.

The Sequence That Keeps Meals Quiet

Meals don't destabilise because of single foods.

They destabilise when energy arrives **too fast, too early**.

The simplest way to prevent that is to let the meal set its pace before energy ramps up.

That's what sequence does.

When slower inputs arrive first, digestion establishes a rhythm the body can manage. Faster foods that come later are absorbed into that rhythm instead of overwhelming it.

The stabilising sequence is straightforward:

Start with foods that take time to break down.
Then move to foods that sustain.
Finish with foods that convert quickly.

This isn't a rule.

It's a default.

You'll notice the difference almost immediately when you try it.

Meals that begin slowly tend to unfold quietly.
Meals that begin quickly tend to compress — even when everything else is reasonable.

The reason is simple: the body doesn't slow mid-meal. Once digestion accelerates, it stays accelerated until the job is done.

Trying to correct a meal after it has already started rarely works. Adding more food doesn't slow the system — it usually gives it more to process at the same speed.

But when the opening is stable, everything downstream behaves differently.

Hunger arrives later.
Cravings soften.
Energy holds.

What makes this powerful is how flexible it is.

The same sequence works with home cooking, restaurant meals, shared plates, and imperfect choices. You're not eliminating anything. You're deciding **what sets the pace.**

Once you start noticing this, eating shifts from restraint to timing.

You stop asking whether a food is "allowed."
You start noticing whether it's setting the speed or riding one.

That change alone removes a surprising amount of effort.

Why This Pattern Feels Familiar

Once you recognise the sequence, it appears everywhere.

Not in diet plans — but in how meals were traditionally structured long before nutrition advice existed.

Across cultures, meals tended to begin slowly.

Something fibrous.

Something textured.
Something that asked the body to start working before dense
energy arrived.

Only after that came richer or faster components.

This wasn't intentional optimisation. It emerged because meals
that unfolded this way simply felt better afterward. They held
longer. They didn't demand constant correction.

Over time, the pattern stuck.

You see it in soups or vegetables before mains.
In starches arriving after, not first.
In sweets coming at the end, not the beginning.

These traditions weren't about virtue.

They were about **pace**.

Modern eating often reverses that order.

Fast foods arrive first.
Refined foods arrive early.
Energy spikes before digestion has stabilised.

What once acted as a buffer is now often missing.

Recognising this removes the sense that you're adopting a
special strategy. You're restoring a pattern that worked because
it matched how the body regulates flow.

That's why this sequence feels intuitive once tried.

It doesn't fight appetite.
It doesn't demand discipline.

It allows digestion to unfold at a speed the body recognises.

TECHNICAL NOTE — What the Body Is Responding To

The body does not regulate meals based on calories or ingredients. It regulates them based on **the rate at which absorbable energy appears in the bloodstream**.

That rate is set early, primarily by **gastric emptying**. The first material to enter the stomach determines how quickly food is released into the small intestine. Bulky, fibrous foods increase viscosity and activate gastric feedback mechanisms that slow this release. Once established, this slower emptying pattern tends to persist for the remainder of the meal.

When gastric emptying is slow, glucose appears in circulation gradually. Intestinal incretin signalling and pancreatic insulin release rise proportionally rather than pre-emptively. Insulin exposure is shorter, satiety signals align with intake, and normal transitions back toward fat use can occur between meals.

When gastric emptying accelerates early—most commonly when refined starches or liquids arrive first—glucose appears rapidly. Incretin and insulin responses escalate sooner and often overshoot actual clearance needs. If fat is present at the same time, digestion slows only after the surge has begun, extending insulin exposure rather than preventing it.

The downstream result is predictable: blood glucose falls quickly after the peak, counter-regulatory hunger signals activate, and appetite returns despite sufficient energy intake. This response is frequently misattributed to behaviour or food choice, but it is driven by **nutrient delivery velocity**.

Meal pacing works because it alters this sequence. By slowing gastric emptying at the start of a meal, it reduces the rate of glucose appearance, shortens insulin exposure, and prevents reactive hunger. The effect is achieved through **physiological sequencing**, not restriction.

The Same Meal, Three Different Results

Consider a familiar fast-food meal:

lettuce and pickles, a beef patty, cheese and sauce, a bun, and chips.

Nothing about the food changes in the examples below.
Only **how it enters the body** does.

Eaten on a plate

The lettuce and pickles are eaten first.
The meat and cheese follow.
The bun and sauce come next.
The chips are finished last.

Digestion opens slowly.
The stomach releases food at a measured pace.
Energy enters circulation gradually rather than all at once.

The meal settles.
Hunger stays quiet.
There is no crash later.

Eaten as a burger with fries

The chips are eaten first.
The burger follows as a single, compressed unit.

Digestion accelerates immediately.
Energy arrives quickly, before the system has time to stabilise.
Everything that follows enters a faster-moving process.

The meal feels filling but unsettled.
Hunger returns sooner than expected.
Energy dips later.

Blended together

Chewing disappears.
Structure disappears.
Everything arrives at once.

Energy enters circulation at maximum speed.
The body is forced into correction rather than regulation.

Fullness comes quickly.
Hunger returns quickly.
The system never settles.

The food did not change.
The quantity did not change.

Same food. Same amount. Different order — different outcome.

Using the Sequence in Real Life

This isn't something you "follow."

It's something you **nudge**.

Modern meals are mixed. Plates are shared. Eating happens at desks, in restaurants, between obligations. Perfect staging isn't realistic — and it isn't required.

What matters is direction, not precision.

When a meal leans toward starting slowly, it tends to hold better. When it leans toward starting fast, it tends to collapse.

That's the only question worth asking.

You don't need to separate foods cleanly.
You don't need strict order.
You don't need to avoid combinations you enjoy.

You're simply giving the body a brief head start before faster energy arrives.

Sometimes that means beginning with the most textured part of the meal.
Sometimes it means eating what requires chewing before what doesn't.
Sometimes it means pausing briefly before moving to denser foods.

Even small shifts count.

A few minutes of slower digestion at the start of a meal can change the entire downstream experience. The system sets its pace early — and once set, it carries through.

That's why this works in imperfect situations.

At restaurants.
At social events.
On busy days with limited options.

You're not fighting the environment.

You're adapting inside it.

Over time, this becomes automatic.

You stop thinking in terms of rules and start noticing outcomes. Meals that hold feel different. Days that stay steady feel different. Eating recedes into the background more often.

That's the goal.

Not to manage food constantly — but to make food demand less attention.

When this sequence is used consistently, many people notice another quiet change: they reach satisfaction sooner than they expect.

Not because they are restraining themselves, but because the system has finished what it needs to do.

At that point, continuing to eat often feels neutral rather than satisfying. The impulse to keep going fades on its own. Portions that once felt normal begin to feel unnecessary — not emotionally, but mechanically.

This is not something to push through. Stopping when appetite quiets preserves stability. Eating past that point usually reintroduces correction, even when the food itself is reasonable.

This is why intake often decreases on its own when rhythm is restored. Signals complete earlier, so eating ends earlier. Nothing is counted. Nothing is withheld.

Some food cultures formalised this long ago. In Japan, eating to comfortable satisfaction rather than finishing the plate is practiced deliberately — not as restraint, but as respect for completion. The goal is not fullness. It is to stop when the system is quiet.

In the next chapter, we'll step back from individual meals and apply the same logic across the week — showing how rhythm between eating and rest days prevents instability from stacking over time.

The principle does not change.

Set the pace correctly, and the system does the rest.

CHAPTER 4 — Why Periodic Eating Pauses Matter

Up to this point, this book has focused on how food enters the body.

Order.
Timing.
Pace.

Those changes alone stabilise appetite, flatten glucose spikes, and reduce the day-to-day volatility most people experience around eating.

So the next question is straightforward:

Why pause eating at all?

If meal timing already improves metabolic stability, what does fasting add?

The answer is not intensity.
It is **maintenance**.

Two operating states, not one

Human metabolism does not operate as a single continuous mode.

It alternates between:

- a **fed state**, where incoming energy is processed

- a **maintenance state**, where repair and recalibration

occur

Eating activates the fed state.
Time without intake allows the maintenance state to run.

When eating is frequent or constant, the second state is shortened or skipped. Not because something is broken, but because the signal to switch never arrives.

Periodic eating pauses exist to restore that signal.

What changes when intake stops

When food is absent for long enough, a predictable sequence unfolds.

Insulin falls.
Stored energy becomes accessible.
Repair processes that are suppressed during feeding resume.

Damaged proteins are recycled.
Old cellular components are broken down.
Mitochondrial function is refreshed.
Inflammatory signalling quiets.

This is not an emergency response.
It is routine background work.

The body performs this maintenance when conditions allow it.
A short, planned eating pause creates those conditions.

Why this matters even without weight loss

These maintenance processes are associated with:

- preserved insulin sensitivity

- lower baseline inflammation

- improved metabolic flexibility

- more stable appetite signalling over time

- steadier vascular and pressure regulation over time

None of these require visible weight change to be meaningful.

Weight loss may occur for some people.
For others, it does not.

Neither outcome determines whether the process is working.

The goal here is **metabolic stability**, not scale movement.

When an Eating Pause Helps — and When It Doesn't Yet

Eating pauses only work cleanly once the system is stable enough to use them.

This matters, because many people reach for fasting at exactly the moment their body is still correcting constantly. In that state, removing food does not create rest — it creates another transition the system has to manage.

A pause supports maintenance when insulin is already falling between meals, hunger arrives predictably rather than urgently, and energy holds without constant input. In that state, the system can stand down. Repair resumes quietly. Signals resolve instead of stacking.

When those conditions are not present, the same pause can feel noisy or stressful — not because fasting is harmful, but because the body is still compensating for instability created earlier.

This is why fasting often:

- works once, then feels harder each time,

- produces fatigue instead of clarity,

- or feels like a test rather than relief.

The issue is not the pause itself.
It is when it is introduced.

The first layer of this method — meal pacing — exists specifically to prepare the system for rest. By slowing the opening of digestion and reducing correction load, pacing allows energy to arrive and clear cleanly. Hunger softens. Meals begin to hold. The body finishes what it starts.

If daily meals are still destabilising, skipping them simply removes support while instability remains. That is not a failure. It is a sequencing issue.

Most people don't need to decide when to fast. Readiness usually appears on its own. Meals hold longer. Hunger arrives later. Gaps between eating feel tolerable. Often, people find themselves pausing intake without planning to — not because they are trying, but because the body is no longer asking.

That is the signal this method respects.

If you are currently dealing with active medical concerns — such as unstable blood pressure, poorly controlled blood sugar, significant anxiety, or sleep disruption — the weekly eating pauses described next are not the place to start. That does not mean this method isn't for you. It means the order matters.

In these situations, the pacing layer introduced earlier is the correct focus. Slowing how meals begin, reducing signal overload, and allowing digestion to complete often stabilise the system enough for improvement to begin — without removing food.

If you are already under medical care for blood pressure, blood sugar, or other metabolic concerns, it is sensible to let your clinician know before applying the weekly eating pauses described next. Not because the method is extreme, but because changing eating rhythm can alter signals your care may already be addressing.

The daily pacing layer does not usually require this step.
The weekly pause sometimes does.

This book does not ask you to push through warning signs.
It asks you to change conditions until those signs no longer appear.

Duration matters, but extremes are unnecessary

Once the system is prepared, very little absence is needed to trigger maintenance.

Longer fasts are sometimes discussed as if they are required for benefit.

They are not.

The body does not reward hardship.
It responds to signals.

A finite eating pause that is long enough to:

- lower insulin

- allow repair processes to complete

- recalibrate appetite expectation

is sufficient when repeated consistently.

Beyond that point, returns diminish while cost increases.

This method deliberately avoids escalation.

The fast is rarely the problem

When people struggle with fasting, the issue is almost never the pause itself.

It is the **entry**.

If the body enters an eating pause after:

- high sugar intake

- refined carbohydrates

- constant grazing

then insulin remains elevated and the transition is noisy.

If the day before the pause is:

- free of sugar

- free of refined carbohydrates

- paced and calm

then insulin begins falling before the pause even starts.

In that state, the eating pause is quiet and predictable.

This is why structure before the fast matters more than willpower during it.

A rhythm, not a challenge

The fasting rhythm introduced next is:

- limited in duration

- capped in depth

- designed to be repeated indefinitely

There is no ladder to climb.
There is no benefit to pushing further.
There is no expectation of progression.

The value comes from **repeatability**, not intensity.

A system that can be followed calmly for years produces more benefit than one that requires constant effort or optimisation.

How to read what follows

The weekly rhythm that follows is not presented as an upgrade or a test.

It is simply the **simplest structure** that reliably creates a maintenance window without disrupting daily life.

Read it as architecture.

The rules exist to keep the system quiet, not to challenge you.

CHAPTER 5 — Why Weeks Matter More Than Days

Most people try to improve their health one day at a time.

They have a good day, followed by a worse one.
They eat carefully, then drift.
They reset, then repeat.

When this happens, it is easy to assume the issue is discipline, consistency, or motivation.

It isn't.

The problem is scale.

Daily behaviour is noisy

At the daily level, the body is constantly responding to short-term input.

Meals arrive.
Energy rises.
Signals fluctuate.
Hunger appears and fades.

Even when meals are well structured, the body is still processing *what just happened.*
The system never has enough distance to evaluate the pattern as a whole.

This is why individual "good days" often fail to produce lasting change.

They are absorbed by the noise of the system.

Instability stacks quietly

When intake is inconsistent, the effects do not cancel out.
They accumulate.

Small excesses do not resolve overnight.
Shortfalls do not disappear by morning.

Instead, the body carries forward:

- incomplete recovery

- unresolved signalling

- lingering inflammatory load

- distorted appetite expectation

None of this feels dramatic in the moment.

It feels like:

- vague hunger

- low-grade fatigue

- unpredictable cravings

- difficulty reading true appetite

This is not failure.
It is delayed accounting.

The body responds to patterns, not intentions

Biological systems do not respond to effort or resolve.

They respond to **repetition**.

A single calm day does not establish a signal.
A repeated rhythm does.

This is why stability rarely emerges from isolated changes, no matter how well executed they are.

The body is not asking:

> "Was today good?"

It is asking:

> "What usually happens?"

Contrast is required for clarity

Stability does not come from sameness.

It comes from **contrast**.

When input never changes, signals blur.
When contrast appears, the system can recalibrate.

Importantly, the contrast does not need to be extreme.
It needs to be **predictable**.

Unpredictable contrast creates stress.
Predictable contrast creates regulation.

This is a critical distinction.

Why weeks are the correct unit

A week is long enough for:

- signals to rise and fall

- recovery to complete

- expectation to reset

- cumulative effects to become visible

It is also short enough to:

- remain legible

- repeat without effort

- integrate into real life

Daily variation disappears at the weekly level.
Patterns become obvious.

This is why systems designed around weeks succeed where daily fixes fail.

Effort decreases when structure is external

When structure exists at the weekly level, individual days carry less weight.

There is no need to:

- correct every deviation

- perfect every meal

- interpret every signal

The system absorbs small variations automatically.

This reduces effort not by lowering standards, but by **removing constant decision-making**.

The body responds well to this.

So do people.

Why predictability matters more than intensity

Intense contrast creates reaction.
Predictable contrast creates adaptation.

A system that relies on intensity:

- demands motivation

- invites escalation

- eventually breaks

A system built on predictability:

- runs quietly

- requires little attention

- compounds over time

The goal here is not disruption.

It is **maintenance**.

What this chapter establishes

This chapter is not about rules.

It establishes three principles that everything that follows
depends on:

1. Stability emerges from patterns, not days

2. Contrast works when it is predictable

3. Weeks are the smallest unit where this reliably happens

Nothing has been implemented yet.
Nothing has been prescribed.

Only the scale has been set.

What comes next

Within a weekly rhythm, contrast must still take a form.

The next chapter explains **why periodic pauses in intake are
the quietest and most reliable way to create that contrast—**
without escalation, without intensity, and without disruption.

Read it as continuation, not instruction.

The structure comes before the mechanism.

CHAPTER 6 — The Default Week

A Note on Feeding Patterns

Human metabolism is not built around constant intake.

It is built for **variability**.

For most of human history, eating did not occur at fixed intervals or in uniform daily patterns. Food availability changed with weather, travel, success, and circumstance. As a result, the body evolved systems that could shift smoothly between feeding and non-feeding states without loss of function.

This flexibility is not a stress response.
It is a normal operating mode.

When food is absent for a time, insulin levels fall, stored energy becomes available, and hunger rises and falls in waves rather than increasing indefinitely. When food returns, digestion resumes without damage or confusion. The system is designed to move between these states.

What the body is less well suited for is **continuous intake**.

When eating happens frequently and without pause, digestion never fully completes. Signals overlap. Fuel switching is delayed. Hunger becomes less predictable — not because the body needs more food, but because it hasn't had space to finish processing what already arrived.

This is why introducing **contrast** matters.

Not because fasting is required.
Not because eating less is superior.

But because periods of relative quiet allow appetite and metabolism to complete cycles that constant intake keeps interrupting.

The structure introduced in this chapter uses that principle deliberately — not as a demand, but as a tool. It creates enough difference between days for the system to settle, while keeping eating days normal, social, and complete.

Nothing here assumes a specific meal frequency.
Nothing requires skipping meals forever.

It simply restores a pattern the body already knows how to handle.

Why This Fits the Modern Week

The seven-day week is not a metabolic construct.

It is a social one.

Work schedules, school timetables, shared days off, religious traditions, and commerce have all shaped the modern week into a repeating unit of effort and rest. Eating patterns were eventually pulled into that structure — not because the body required it, but because coordination did.

The body responds to difference between periods of intake and periods of quiet. The calendar simply provides a convenient container for that contrast to occur without constant decision-making.

This is why the approach outlined in this chapter works within an ordinary week instead of asking you to escape it.

What Quiet Days Actually Do

When intake pauses for long enough, the body shifts state.

This is not a special mode or a stress response. It is a normal transition the system is designed to make when food stops arriving.

As digestion completes, insulin levels fall. With less incoming energy to manage, the body begins drawing on stored fuel instead of circulating glucose. Fat becomes the primary source, not all at once, but progressively as the quiet period continues.

This shift takes time.

Early in a fast, the body is finishing recent work — clearing glucose, emptying glycogen, resolving signals that were already in motion. Only after that does sustained fat use become dominant. The longer the quiet lasts, the deeper that process runs.

This is why short pauses feel different from longer ones.

Both reduce noise.
Only longer ones create a clear reset signal.

As insulin remains low for longer stretches, sensitivity improves — not because insulin is avoided, but because it is no longer held elevated all day. When eating resumes, the system responds more efficiently. Signals rise and fall cleanly instead of lingering.

None of this requires constant fasting.

It requires **contrast**.

Meal pacing creates contrast within a meal.
Longer pauses create contrast across days.

That is the entire method.

Quiet days are not about eating less forever. They are about giving metabolism enough uninterrupted time to complete cycles that constant intake keeps restarting.

The structure that follows simply uses the week as a convenient container for that process.

Rather than eating identically every day — or requiring strict adherence to irregular schedules — the method uses the existing rhythm of the week to create variation the body recognises.

Some days are fuller.
Some days are quieter.

Not because one is "better," but because the difference between them allows signals to resolve.

The specific day choices that follow are not rules or mandates.
They are **anchors** — points of stability chosen for practical reasons: predictability, social compatibility, and recovery.
Chosen to meet the week calmly and fit social windows.

They can be moved if needed.
They can be adapted.

What matters is that the pattern creates enough separation for the system to finish its work before the cycle repeats and you understand the consequences of shifting the pattern.

A Shape to Test, Not a Promise to Keep

Up to this point, the focus has been on **why** appetite behaves the way it does.

This chapter gives that understanding a shape you can actually live inside.

Not a rule set.
Not a commitment.
Not something you have to defend or maintain perfectly.

Just a starting rhythm.

Most people don't fail because they chose the wrong approach. They fail because they were handed something that demanded immediate belief, constant precision, or long-term loyalty before their body had a chance to respond.

This is different.

The default week is not something you "adopt."
It's something you **observe**.

Its only purpose is to introduce enough contrast that appetite has space to settle — while keeping eating days comfortable and normal.

Nothing here requires willpower.
Nothing here depends on streaks.
Nothing here assumes ideal weeks.

You're not locking anything in.

You're simply giving your system a week that isn't flat.

Once you've experienced that difference, decisions stop being theoretical.

Why Weeks Matter More Than Individual Days

Most people think in terms of days.

A good day.
A bad day.
A reset tomorrow.

But appetite doesn't operate in 24-hour units.

It carries momentum.

When days are similar — frequent intake, constant correction — signals overlap. Hunger never fully resolves. Even reasonable meals begin to feel demanding.

This is why people can eat well for days and still feel off.

The issue isn't effort.
It's that the system never finishes one cycle before the next begins.

Weeks work better when they contain a pause.

Not extremes.
Not punishment.
Just clear differences between days that are meant for eating and days that are meant for quiet.

When that contrast exists, appetite stops stacking. Hunger becomes predictable instead of reactive. Eating days feel easier because quieter days actually clear signals.

The default week exists to create that contrast without disrupting life.

The Two Kinds of Days

The default week contains two distinct kinds of days.

Eating days, and
Quieter days.

They are not opposites. They support each other.

A brief but important boundary:

If food restriction has ever been a source of distress, loss of control, or obsessive behaviour for you, this structure should be approached with care — or not used at all without support.

The aim here is to reduce friction and restore calm, not to test endurance or suppress appetite. Any approach that increases anxiety around eating is a signal to pause, not push.

Eating Days

Eating days are not restraint days.

They are days where meals are allowed to feel **complete**.

You eat paced meals until satisfied — not cautiously, not partially, not with the sense that you should stop early. These days are meant to feel socially normal. Meals with others fit here.

Enjoyment fits here.

Their job is to finish appetite cleanly.

When eating days do their job, hunger does not linger into the next day looking for resolution.

Quieter Days

Quieter days are not endurance tests.

They are days where intake is low enough — and simple enough — that appetite signals are allowed to rise and fall without constant interruption.

These days are not about fighting hunger.

They're about **not constantly restarting digestion**.

When eating is spread out in small interruptions, hunger never settles. When the day is allowed to stay quiet, appetite peaks and then softens on its own.

The contrast between these two day types is what stabilises the week.

Not intensity.
Not perfection.
Just clarity.

Why Salt Matters on Quieter Days

On quieter days, something subtle but important changes.

As intake drops and insulin stays low, the body begins releasing stored water and sodium. In physiological terms, this is an electrolyte shift: sodium is the primary driver of fluid balance when insulin falls. Because little to no food is coming in on quieter days, that sodium is not being replaced through meals. This is a normal response to reduced eating, not a problem to push through. But if sodium is not replaced, the day can feel harder than it needs to. Water loss increases alongside sodium loss, which means hydration often needs to be more intentional on these days. If you're feeling thirsty, drink.

This loss doesn't show up as hunger.

It shows up as headaches, lightheadedness, fatigue, feeling cold, or a flat, agitated kind of discomfort that doesn't improve with time. These signals are often misread as "low energy" or lack of will — when they're simply signs of depletion.

Warm, salty fluids help because they replace what's being lost without restarting digestion. Light broths, clean miso, or lightly salted drinks support circulation and nerve signalling while keeping the day quiet. I enjoy adding a pinch of salt to my soda water bottle — it tastes wonderful.

This advice doesn't contradict the usual "eat less salt" messaging. That guidance assumes frequent eating and consistently elevated insulin. Quieter days create a different state — one where electrolyte loss increases and replacement becomes supportive rather than excessive.

Used this way, salt isn't stimulation or indulgence.

It's maintenance.

Important Information: If you are managing diagnosed high blood pressure, kidney disease, heart failure, or are taking medications that affect fluid or electrolyte balance, it's sensible to involve a clinician when changing eating patterns.

This isn't because the structure is extreme — it's because these conditions alter how the body handles sodium, fluid, and fasting states.

How to Make Quieter Days Actually Quiet

Quieter days only work if they stay uncomplicated.

The most common mistake is filling them with small inputs.

A bite here.
A drink with calories there.
Something "just to take the edge off."

Each interruption restarts the process and delays resolution. The day feels harder than it needs to be — not because hunger is intense, but because it never gets to finish its cycle.

A calm quieter day has fewer decisions, not more.

Eating, if it happens, is deliberate and contained — not negotiated all day long. Hydration is normal. Activity is normal. Life continues.

What changes is that food stops being central.

When this is done correctly, hunger changes character.

It becomes less urgent.
Less distracting.

Easier to coexist with normal activity.

Energy often feels steadier than expected. Mental noise around food drops faster than anticipated.

This isn't something you push through.

If a quieter day feels agitating, it usually means too much is happening — not too little.

Letting Eating Days Do Their Job

The rhythm only holds if eating days are allowed to work.

If eating days become cautious — trimmed portions, delayed meals, half-satisfaction — they stop supporting the system. Hunger never fully resolves, and quieter days end up carrying work they weren't designed for.

That's when the week becomes fragile.

Eating days are not rewards.
They are not compensation.

They are **stability days**.

Their job is to allow appetite to complete so that quieter days don't have to manage unfinished signals.

When eating days are clean and complete, something important happens:

- Cravings don't stack

- Snacking fades

- The week stops oscillating

Planning also simplifies.

Instead of asking, "Should I eat this?"
You ask, "What kind of day is this?"

That single distinction removes a large amount of mental effort.

Over time, the body learns the rhythm. Appetite anticipates space. Hunger stops escalating unnecessarily. Eating becomes less emotionally charged.

When the Week Breaks

No week goes exactly to plan.

Meals run long.
Events appear.
Quieter days get interrupted.

This method assumes that.

What matters is not precision — it's **returning to contrast**.

Missing a quieter day doesn't collapse the system.
An extra eating day doesn't undo progress.
A disrupted week doesn't require a reset.

The mistake is treating disruption as failure.

That response creates more instability than the disruption itself.

A better approach is simpler.

When the rhythm breaks, you don't compensate.

You don't restrict harder.
You don't try to erase what happened.

You just restore clarity.

That might mean letting the next quieter day stay genuinely quiet.
Or letting the next eating day be fully complete instead of cautious.
Or simply re-establishing the distinction between day types.

The system doesn't need correction.
It needs room.

Once contrast returns, appetite settles quickly. The sense of being "off" fades without force.

This is why the default week is resilient.

It doesn't rely on streaks.
It doesn't punish imperfection.
It recovers naturally.

What Comes Next

Up to this point, we've been describing **why rhythm works**, not how to optimise it.

That distinction matters.

A rhythm that only functions when conditions are perfect is fragile.
A rhythm that works under ordinary life pressure is resilient.

The purpose of the quieter days described here is not to create extremes, nor to force outcomes. It is to introduce **predictable contrast** into the week so that signals are allowed to resolve before the next cycle begins.

What remains is to show how that contrast is placed.

Not expanded.
Not intensified.
Placed.

The next chapter explains why **a limited, periodic pause in intake** is the simplest and most reliable way to create this contrast — and why it is intentionally capped rather than extended.

Read it as clarification, not escalation.

The aim is not to do more.

It is to do **just enough**, consistently, so that the week carries its own stability without constant effort.

CHAPTER 7 — Why Weight Loss Follows Stability

What Changes When the System Calms

Up to this point, the focus has been appetite — not weight.

That choice is deliberate.

Most approaches attempt to change weight directly: eat less, burn more, push harder. When results slow, effort increases. Hunger becomes something to manage, and progress depends on restraint.

This method works differently.

It stabilises the system that determines how much effort is required in the first place.

When appetite is unstable, weight loss feels like work. Hunger intrudes. Cravings interrupt. Decisions accumulate. Progress requires constant correction.

When appetite stabilises, the context changes.

Eating quietens.
Portions feel proportionate.
Recovery between meals improves.

Not because weight loss is being pursued — but because the body is no longer reacting to repeated spikes and compensations.

In an unstable state, the body behaves defensively. Energy is conserved. Drops are corrected aggressively. Weight loss becomes harder the more it is forced.

Stability removes that defence.

When energy arrives at a manageable pace and clears fully between eating events, the system stops overcorrecting. Hunger softens. Intake adjusts without pressure.

When weight loss occurs in this state, it does so quietly — not through restriction, but through fewer reactive eating moments across the week.

This is why many people notice change only after they stop chasing it.

What Progress Actually Looks Like

When appetite begins to stabilise, weight rarely changes immediately.

That can feel uncomfortable.

Many people have been conditioned to expect rapid movement as proof that something is working. A quick drop reassures. A slower response creates doubt.

Stability does not announce itself dramatically.

It shows up as **less noise.**

Fewer urges to correct.
Fewer swings in intake.
Fewer moments where food feels urgent.

These shifts often appear before any visible change on the scale.

This is not a stall.
It is recalibration.

After long periods of instability, the body does not immediately release reserves when conditions improve. Early on, it observes. Signals soften before storage adjusts.

If pressure is added during this phase — by tightening eating days, shrinking portions, or adding extra quiet days — the system often re-enters defence mode. Hunger sharpens. Cravings return. Effort increases.

This is why many attempts fail just as they begin to "work."

The order matters.

Eating feels easier before it looks lighter.
Weeks feel calmer before weight moves.
Effort drops before results accumulate.

When change comes, it often arrives in steps.

A shift.
A pause.
Another shift.

That pattern reflects adaptation, not inconsistency.

The correct instruction during this phase is simple:

Hold the structure steady.

Signals That Matter More Than the Scale

Weight is a lagging indicator.

Stability appears elsewhere first.

One of the earliest changes is **timing**.

Hunger arrives later. Meals hold longer. Gaps between eating events extend without effort. Delays occur naturally, not through restraint.

Another change is **quality**.

Hunger feels less sharp and less urgent. It can be noticed without immediate response. This is not suppression — it is resolution.

Mental load often decreases.

Food decisions feel lighter. Eating occupies less background attention. The constant negotiation fades.

Energy tends to smooth out.

Fewer afternoon drops.
Less reliance on quick fixes.
More even focus across the day.

Sleep and mood often improve before weight changes. These are not side effects. They are indicators that the system is no longer cycling aggressively.

When these signals improve, weight loss is usually **pending**, not blocked.

The most common mistake at this point is interference.

If these signs are present, the correct response is to change nothing.

Why Acceleration Backfires

When weight begins to move, the urge to accelerate is strong.

Feedback appears.
Clothes fit differently.
Momentum feels fragile.

The instinct follows: if this is working, push it.

This is where many systems fail.

Acceleration reintroduces instability.

Eating days become cautious.
Quieter days multiply.
Portions shrink on top of a structure that was already sufficient.

The result is predictable.

Hunger sharpens.
Cravings return.
Effort increases.

The system that allowed weight to change was a stable one.
When conditions shift too quickly, the body responds defensively
— even when the intent is healthy.

Weight loss that lasts is not held by pressure.

It is held by **continuity**.

If progress slows, the answer is rarely to tighten immediately.

It is to check for drift.

Have eating days become incomplete?

Have quiet periods fragmented?
Has grazing crept back in?

Most stalls come from erosion of contrast, not insufficiency.

Restoring clarity restores momentum.

The discipline here is not restriction.

It is restraint from interference.

When Weight Stops Being a Project

Many systems treat maintenance as a separate phase.

Weight is lost through effort, then held through vigilance. This framing creates anxiety. People assume hunger will return once active effort stops.

Stability dissolves that divide.

When weight loss occurs as a downstream effect of calm appetite and clear rhythm, there is no sharp transition into maintenance. The same structure that allowed change is the structure that allows it to settle.

Nothing new is required.

Eating days remain complete.
Quieter days continue to create space.
Meals stay paced without thought.

At some point, weight stops changing.

Not because effort dropped — but because the body reached a place it is comfortable holding under stable conditions.

That pause is not failure.

It is resolution.

Forcing further loss at this point often reintroduces instability and reverses progress, not because the body is resistant, but because the rhythm was disturbed.

A stable system does not require vigilance.

It self-regulates.

Maintenance, in this context, is not something you do.

It is what happens when the structure remains intact.

Food stops feeling like a project.
Weight stops feeling precarious.
The week supports itself.

That is the real outcome of the method — not a number to defend, but the absence of struggle.

CHAPTER 8 — When Things Don't Behave as Expected

Why "Problems" Usually Aren't Problems

At some point, almost everyone reaches a moment of uncertainty.

Hunger shows up earlier than expected.
A quieter day feels harder than usual.
Weight pauses, or shifts in a direction you didn't anticipate.

The reflex is immediate:

Something must be wrong.

This chapter exists to slow that reaction down.

Because in most cases, nothing has broken.

When a system has been unstable for a long time, it doesn't respond to change in a straight line. Signals surface unevenly. Old patterns reappear briefly. The body tests whether new conditions will hold.

That testing can look like regression if you don't expect it.

But it isn't.

Most issues people encounter at this stage fall into one of three categories:

- the system is still settling

- contrast has softened without being noticed

- expectations have moved faster than physiology

None of these require force.

They require interpretation.

Troubleshooting in this method is not about tightening control. It's about identifying **where stability was interrupted** — often in small, ordinary ways.

A quieter day that became fragmented.
An eating day that stopped being complete.
A week that lost contrast due to stress or busyness.

These are not discipline failures.

They are normal fluctuations in a system learning a new rhythm.

The mistake is treating every deviation as proof the method doesn't work. That reaction leads back to familiar habits: doing more, restricting harder, or abandoning structure entirely.

Instead of asking, *"What did I do wrong?"*
This chapter asks, *"What signal is the system sending?"*

Once you learn to read those signals, most issues resolve with small adjustments — often by removing interference rather than adding effort.

When Hunger Shows Up Earlier Than You Thought

One of the first concerns people raise is this:

"I'm following the sequence. I'm using the rhythm. But I'm still getting hungry earlier than I expected."

This can feel discouraging if you assumed hunger would simply quiet and stay quiet.

What's happening here is usually **timing**, not failure.

When the system has spent years responding to frequent intake and fast energy, its signals are calibrated to expect regular correction. Early hunger is often the echo of that expectation — not evidence that something is wrong.

The signal arrives on the old schedule, even though the conditions have changed.

This is common in the early weeks.

The body checks.
It looks for the usual response.
When food doesn't arrive immediately, hunger appears briefly to see if it still works.

If the system is stable, that signal often fades on its own.

This is where interpretation matters.

If early hunger is treated as a command, the old cycle restarts.
If it's treated as information, the system adjusts.

There is a useful distinction to notice.

Urgent hunger escalates quickly. It demands action. It's often tied to a crash or correction.
Residual hunger is quieter. It appears, lingers lightly, and passes if it isn't constantly interrupted.

Most early hunger in a stabilising system is residual.

If energy is steady, mood is even, and focus is intact, the signal is usually transitional. The system is updating its expectations.

In those cases, the most effective response is often to **do nothing** — briefly — and observe.

Not indefinitely.
Just long enough to see whether the signal resolves.

When hunger completes its cycle without escalation, the body learns something important: it no longer needs to raise volume as quickly.

That learning compounds.

Over days and weeks, hunger arrives later — not because it's suppressed, but because the system has recalibrated.

Early hunger is not a reason to intervene.

It's often a reason to hold the structure steady.

When Quieter Days Feel Harder Than Expected

Another concern appears once the weekly rhythm is in place:

"Eating days feel fine, but quieter days are harder than I expected."

Difficulty alone doesn't indicate a problem.

Quieter days can feel hard for two very different reasons.

One is **instability**.

The other is **contrast**.

They feel similar on the surface, but they behave differently underneath.

When a quieter day is hard because of instability, hunger escalates quickly. Energy dips. Focus fragments. The day feels like something to endure. This usually points to interference — fragmented eating, frequent small inputs, or an eating day that didn't fully resolve appetite.

In that case, the system is still busy.

But when a quieter day is hard because of contrast, the experience is different.

Hunger appears but doesn't spiral.
Energy remains workable.
The discomfort is noticeable but contained.

For people used to constant input, clear space can feel unfamiliar. The mind interprets that unfamiliarity as difficulty, even when the body is functioning well.

This is why quieter days often feel hardest **before** they feel easier.

The system is learning that it can operate without continuous correction. That learning process isn't silent.

The key distinction is simple:

If the day feels chaotic, something is interrupting resolution.
If the day feels sparse but steady, the system is doing its work.

The mistake is responding to the second case as if it were the first.

Adding inputs to "smooth things out" prevents the day from completing its cycle. The difficulty repeats next time instead of resolving.

A quieter day doesn't need to feel pleasant.

It needs to feel **finite**.

When hunger rises and falls without constant interruption, the body learns that escalation isn't required. That learning reduces future difficulty far more reliably than comfort inputs ever do.

This isn't about pushing through at all costs.

If energy collapses or mood destabilises, that's information. But if the day is simply quiet and unfamiliar, letting it be often produces the fastest adaptation.

When Weight Pauses or Moves the "Wrong" Way

Weight rarely moves in a straight line.

Even when appetite is calmer, meals are holding, and weeks feel stable, the scale can pause — or move upward briefly.

For many people, this is the most destabilising moment.

Everything else feels better, but the number doesn't cooperate.

Weight is a lagging indicator.

It reflects fluid, glycogen, digestion, inflammation, and timing —

all of which change as the system stabilises.

Early on, it's common for weight to pause while appetite improves.

That's not a contradiction.

It's sequencing.

When instability reduces, the body first normalises internal signals. Release often follows later. During that recalibration phase, pushing for faster loss tends to reintroduce defence.

This is why reacting to short-term changes is risky.

Tightening structure in response to a pause often sharpens hunger and increases effort — even when the system was improving.

A better question than "Why isn't the scale moving?" is:

"Is appetite still calmer than it was?"

If hunger is quieter, decisions feel lighter, and weeks feel more stable, the system is still progressing — even if the scale hasn't caught up.

When weight loss follows stability, it often arrives in steps.

A shift.
A pause.
Another shift.

The instruction during a pause is not to intervene.

It's to **hold conditions steady** long enough for internal changes to complete.

When Appetite Comes Back Loudly

Few moments are more unsettling than this:

Things were working.
The week felt calm.
Then appetite suddenly becomes loud again.

This is rarely permanent, and it almost always has a clear cause.

There are three common reasons.

Drift.
Small changes accumulate. Eating days become cautious. Quieter days fragment. Snacks reappear. Contrast softens.

Stress.
Sleep disruption, illness, travel, emotional load, or sustained pressure can temporarily amplify hunger — even when structure remains intact.

Resolution.
As stability holds, stored signals sometimes release in waves. Appetite spikes briefly as the system rebalances, then settles again.

The mistake is responding to any of these with force.

Restriction, compensation, or tightening usually turns a temporary signal into a prolonged one.

The better response starts with one question:

"What changed recently — structurally?"

Not emotionally.

If drift is present, restore roles. Let eating days be complete. Let quieter days be genuinely quiet.

If stress is present, hold the rhythm steady. The structure stabilises load; it isn't meant to be optimised under pressure.

If resolution is underway, patience is the response. Appetite that rises and then falls without intervention teaches the system it doesn't need to escalate next time.

The unifying principle is simple:

Loud appetite is information, not instruction.

Turning Signals Into Guidance

By now, the pattern should be clear.

Most issues are not signs that the method has failed. They're signs that the system is communicating.

Hunger timing.
Appetite intensity.
Energy shifts.
Weight pauses.

None of these require immediate correction.

Instead of asking, *"How do I stop this?"*
You ask, *"What is the system responding to?"*

That shift removes urgency.

Troubleshooting becomes quiet.

You return to fundamentals:

Are eating days complete?
Are quieter days genuinely quiet?
Is contrast still present?
Has life added stress that needs space, not optimisation?

Most of the time, these questions are enough.

If the answers are clear, the system usually settles again on its own. If not, the adjustment is small — restoring a role that drifted, not inventing a new rule.

This is how the method sustains itself.

Not through vigilance.
Not through perfection.
But through **interpretation**.

Once signals stop feeling threatening, eating stops feeling fragile. Life fits inside the rhythm instead of constantly disrupting it.

In the next chapter, we'll move away from troubleshooting and focus on clarifying how the rhythm is supported in everyday situations — simple considerations that help it hold under different pressures without changing its shape.

Nothing here needs to be fixed.

It only needs to be understood.

CHAPTER 9 — The Weekly Rhythm

The Controlled Portion of the Week

Sunday — Entry Day

Sunday functions as an **entry day**.

Its role is not restriction.
Its role is preparation.

The purpose of the entry day is to slow digestion and reduce signal carry-over before the fasting window begins. This is done through food order and composition, not through eating less.

Meals on the entry day are complete and paced.

They prioritise:

- Fibre from vegetables

- Protein as the primary energy source

- Fats in moderate amounts

- Minimal sugar and refined carbohydrates

This reduces volatility going into the fasting window and significantly improves how the absence period feels.

The final meal of Sunday closes eating cleanly.

Once digestion completes, the fasting window begins.

Monday and Tuesday — The Fasting Window

Monday and Tuesday together form a **single, continuous 48-hour fasting window.**

In this book, a *fasting window* refers to a protected period of **complete digestive absence**, beginning after the final meal and ending with a structured re-entry meal.

During the fasting window, the goal is not endurance.

It is **absence.**

Nothing should meaningfully restart digestion.

That means:

- No food

- No liquids containing calories

- No liquids containing fibre

- No liquids containing food particles

This includes items often misunderstood as "safe":

- Broths with vegetable matter

- Miso if it contains solids

- Konjac or fibre-based soups

- Kefir

- Kombucha

- Probiotic drinks

- Any blended or suspended food particles

All of these **reintroduce digestive activity** and shorten the fasting window, even if they feel light.

Water, mineral water, salt, and plain electrolytes that contain no energy or substrate do not meaningfully interrupt absence.

Coffee and tea, if used, should be plain and minimal. Their role is stimulation, not feeding.

The fasting window is not about deprivation.

It is about allowing signals to complete without interruption.

What This Window Is Doing

When digestion is fully absent for long enough, several things happen quietly:

- Insulin remains low and stable

- Hunger signals complete instead of stacking

- Energy shifts away from constant correction

- Appetite volume reduces without effort

These effects are not achieved by force.

They are achieved by **not interfering**.

The most common way people make this window harder than necessary is by trying to soften it with inputs. Even small inputs restart digestion and reset the clock.

Holding the window clean is what makes it tolerable.

Not toughness.

Wednesday — Structured Re-Entry

Wednesday exists for one purpose: **to reintroduce digestion without destabilising appetite.**

The fasting window ends with a deliberate re-entry, not a rebound.

After 48 hours of absence, the digestive system is highly responsive. How food is reintroduced determines whether the benefits of the window carry forward or collapse immediately.

Re-entry meals on Wednesday follow a strict order:

- Acid first

- Fibre from vegetables next

- Protein as the primary intake

- Fats in moderate amounts

- Carbohydrates minimal or absent

This is not about control.

It is about preventing a sudden spike that forces correction.

Meals should be complete, paced, and eaten without urgency. Liquid calories, sugars, and refined carbohydrates at this point tend to overshoot appetite and re-ignite hunger signals prematurely.

If re-entry is handled cleanly, most people notice that hunger remains softer through the day rather than escalating.

That is the signal that the window completed successfully.

Thursday to Saturday — Living Inside the Rhythm

Thursday through Saturday are **not controlled days**.

They are normal eating days that use the food-order principles introduced earlier in the book, but without time restriction.

There is no fasting window here.

There is no requirement to eat less.

There is no requirement to compensate.

The only instruction is **order and completion**.

Meals begin with acid and fibre, move through protein, and end with fats and carbohydrates if desired. Eating is allowed to be social, flexible, and responsive to life.

These days exist to make the structure sustainable.

Without them, the rhythm becomes a project.

With them, it becomes background.

How the Structure Fits Into a Modern Week

Up to this point, the method has focused on *how* eating works — pace, order, and completion.

This chapter introduces *when* those principles are applied across the week.

The weekly rhythm used in this book is designed to fit a modern working life while still allowing the body to experience clear separation between eating and absence. It does not require constant control, and it does not ask you to organise your life around food.

Instead, it places structure where it has the greatest effect and leaves the rest of the week largely intact.

The core rhythm uses **four defined days:**

- A **structured entry day**

- A **48-hour fasting window**

- A **structured re-entry**

- Followed by **unstructured but paced eating days**

Only the first half of the week is controlled.

The second half is lived.

This is deliberate.

Why Only Part of the Week Is Structured

Many systems fail because they demand too much continuity.

They require constant vigilance, constant restraint, or constant optimisation. That works briefly, then collapses.

This method does not attempt to control the entire week.

It places structure where it has the greatest physiological effect and leaves the rest alone.

The fasting window does the work.

The entry and re-entry protect it.

The remaining days allow life to continue without friction.

This balance is what makes the rhythm repeatable.

Health Before Weight Loss

For many readers, the goal of this structure is **health, stability, and longevity**, not aggressive fat loss.

A single 48-hour fasting window per week is sufficient to:

- Reduce insulin volatility

- Improve appetite signalling

- Increase metabolic flexibility

- Lower background inflammation over time

These benefits emerge **without** extended deprivation and without needing to escalate the protocol.

Weight loss may occur.

But it is not forced.

It follows the same pattern described earlier: appetite calms first, effort drops second, and visible change appears later.

For those who want a more weight-loss-focused application, the method can be extended.

That option is addressed separately.

Holding the Structure

The success of this rhythm depends less on precision than on **clarity**.

When the entry day is clean, the fasting window is protected, and re-entry is paced, the rest of the week tends to organise itself.

If something feels harder over time, the answer is rarely to push further.

It is usually to check whether the window is being interrupted, softened, or fragmented.

Stability comes from protection, not pressure.

What Comes Next

With the weekly rhythm established, the next chapters will explore:

- How the structure can be moved to different parts of the week
- How to live with it across changing schedules
- How to adapt it without losing its effect

For readers whose primary goal is weight loss rather than health maintenance, a separate application is provided next.

It uses the same principles — not more force.

CHAPTER 10 — How Eating Days Stay Invisible

Eating days in this system are not there to refuel aggressively.

They are there to **not interrupt fat burning**.

This is the mistake most people make.

They fast correctly — then unknowingly restart appetite, insulin, and reward cycles the moment food returns. Not because of food choice, but because of **arrival speed**.

Food that arrives slowly keeps the system calm.
Food that arrives fast reactivates defence.

What matters on eating days is not what you eat.

It is **how signals arrive**.

That is why the sequence exists.

The Only Sequence That Matters

Every eating day in Part 2 follows the same internal order.

Not as a rule — as physics.

1. **Acid**

2. **Fibre**

3. **Pause**

4. **Protein**

5. **Pause**

6. **Fat**

7. **Carbohydrate (if used)**

8. **Long pause before dessert or substitutes**

This order keeps insulin suppressed, digestion slow, and appetite quiet.

Reverse it, and the week becomes noisy.

Acid Comes First — Always

Acid slows gastric emptying.

That single effect shapes the entire meal.

When acid arrives first, everything that follows enters the bloodstream more gradually. Insulin rises slower. Hunger rebound weakens.

This is why a small amount of acid before eating changes the entire outcome.

Typical forms:

- diluted apple cider vinegar

- citrus water

- vinegar-based dressings

- fermented vegetable brine

This is not about fat burning.

It is about **tempo control**.

When acid is tolerated, it is used.
When it is not, the rest of the sequence becomes more important.

Fibre Is the Brake

Fibre is not a nutrient here.

It is **structure**.

Taken before calories, fibre creates viscosity and volume. It slows absorption and reduces how aggressively the body responds to what follows.

Effective forms are simple:

- psyllium

- chia gel

- glucomannan

- non-starchy vegetables

After fibre, there is a deliberate pause.

Not long.
Not symbolic.
Just enough for the brake to engage.

Without the pause, fibre does nothing.

This step alone often reduces intake without effort — not by fullness, but by preventing escalation.

Protein Stabilises the System

Protein arrives next, before energy density.

Its job is not muscle building.

Its job is **appetite quieting**.

Protein triggers satiety signalling before fats or carbohydrates appear. That signal prevents later overeating.

Protein can be whole food, or — when appropriate —:

- clean protein powders
- unsweetened strained yoghurt

These are tools, not snacks.

Protein always follows fibre.
Protein never follows sugar.

After protein, there is another short pause.

This pause is where restraint disappears.

The body decides for you how much comes next.

Fat Is Functional, Not Primary

Fat is present — but it is not foregrounded.

On Sunday and Wednesday, dietary fat competes directly with body fat use. When fat is excessive, fat loss stalls quietly.

So fat is used for:

- flavour

- satisfaction

- absorption

Not for energy loading.

This is why:

- oils are measured

- cream is restrained

- "fat-forward" eating is excluded on these days

Fat makes food livable.
It does not lead the meal.

Carbohydrates Always Arrive Last

Carbohydrates are not forbidden.

They are **sequenced**.

When carbs arrive last:

- insulin response is slower

- glucose peaks are lower

- hunger rebound is muted

When carbs arrive first, even "healthy" ones:

- appetite escalates

- digestion accelerates

- intake increases

This is why people fail on good food.

Order beats intention.

On Sunday and Wednesday, carbohydrates are minimal and
structural.
On Saturday, they are unrestricted.

But they are **always last**.

Dessert Is Delayed, Not Denied

Dessert does not fail this system.

Stacking does.

A long pause — usually one to two hours — separates the meal
from dessert. This allows digestion to complete before anything
sweet arrives, preventing glucose layering and reward escalation.

For most people, time alone is enough.

If dessert still feels abrupt when it arrives, a small fibrous buffer
beforehand can help — something simple and neutral that slows
entry without reopening appetite. This isn't required. It's a
support, used only when needed.

When dessert is desired without restarting hunger loops,
substitutes work well:

- vanilla cream bases with sugar-free protein

- gelatin or chia puddings

- thick unsweetened yoghurt with flavour

These provide closure without reopening appetite.

Dessert is not moralised here.

It is timed.

How This Looks on Each Eating Day

Sunday
Quiet, clearing, preparatory.
Acid and fibre matter most.
Protein leads.
Fat is modest.
Carbs are residual.

Wednesday
Refeed without wake-up.
Sequence is strict.
Fat remains secondary.
Carbs are minimal.

Thursday and Friday
Normal eating days.
No special structure beyond what you've already learned.
Sequence is still followed, but without emphasis or correction.
These days exist to live normally while the system remains quiet.

Saturday
Abundant, social, unrestricted.
Sequence is optional — but powerful if appetite matters.

Saturday works because the rest of the week is silent.

What Happens When the Sequence Is Ignored

When meals begin with sugar, refined starch, or fat-carb combinations, the outcome is predictable:

- rapid digestion

- insulin spikes

- hunger rebound

- increased intake

This is not a willpower failure.

It is eating **without brakes**.

The sequence installs brakes automatically.

Why This Replaces Tracking

Macros describe content.

Sequencing determines **experience**.

Two meals with identical macros can produce opposite days depending on order.

That is why tracking fails long-term.

The body does not respond to spreadsheets.

It responds to **arrival speed**.

Once sequence becomes automatic, eating days stop interfering with fasting days — and fat burning stays on without effort.

That is the point.

CHAPTER 11 — Breaking the Fast Without Breaking the Reset

Breaking a fast is where most people undo their progress.

Not loudly.
Not immediately.
And not in a way that feels like failure.

The damage usually shows up later — as louder hunger, harder fasting, and a sense that the method has suddenly stopped working.

It hasn't.

The re-entry was rushed.

What the Fast Leaves Behind

By the end of a proper fast, several conditions are in place:

- insulin is suppressed

- fat oxidation is dominant

- hunger signalling is minimal

- food expectation has dropped

This is not a fragile state — but it **is responsive.**

The body is quiet, alert, and highly sensitive to input.

What you do next determines whether that state:

- extends naturally, or

- collapses immediately

Most people assume the fast does the work.

In reality, **the re-entry decides how long the work lasts**.

Why Refeeds Fail Even When Food Is "Clean"

Refeeds usually fail for one reason: **speed**.

After fasting, digestion restarts aggressively if food arrives too quickly. Insulin rises faster than it needs to. Appetite circuits wake before satiety has time to register.

This happens even with good food.

Clean ingredients do not protect against fast signals.

Three mistakes account for almost all failed refeeds.

The Three Quiet Ways the Reset Gets Undone

1. Speed

Eating immediately, without buffering, creates a sharp insulin response.

The consequences are delayed, not instant:

- hunger returns the same day

- appetite feels noisier

- the next fast feels heavier

This is often misread as "fasting doesn't work for me."

In reality, the fast worked — it just wasn't allowed to finish.

2. Order

Leading with carbohydrates or fats wakes reward and energy systems before satiety has engaged.

Common examples:

- yoghurt with fruit
- smoothies
- bread or starch "just to start"

The body does not care about intent.

It responds to **arrival order**.

Once reward signalling is active, appetite escalates whether you planned it or not.

3. Density

High fat intake immediately after fasting replaces body-fat use with dietary fat use.

This does not feel wrong.

It feels comfortable — and that's the problem.

The cost appears later as:

- stalled fat loss

- returning hunger

- reduced depth of future fasts

Why this Same Sequence Matters More After Fasting

The sequence used is not new. It's the same pacing principle introduced earlier — applied in a more sensitive state. After fasting, the system responds faster, which makes order and pauses matter more, not less.

The Only Re-Entry That Preserves the Reset

Breaking the fast uses the **same sequence as eating days** — but more carefully.

This is not complexity.

It is restraint from escalation.

Step 1 — Acid First

Before calories return, acid slows everything that follows.

This may be:

- diluted apple cider vinegar

- lemon water

- fermented brine

This step matters **more here than anywhere else** in the week.

It reduces the shock of re-entry.

Step 2 — Fibre Before Energy

The first calories are fibre — not protein, not fat.

Options are simple:

- psyllium

- chia gel

- fibrous vegetables

Then wait.

This pause allows digestion to engage **without stimulation**.

Without this step, everything that follows hits too fast.

Step 3 — Protein Alone

Protein is the first true energy input.

Its role here is not nutrition.

It is **signal control**.

Protein:

- triggers satiety

- blunts rebound hunger

- prepares the system for further intake

Protein powders or yogurt are acceptable here **only** when:

- they are unsweetened

- they are not combined with fats or sugars

After protein, wait again.

These pauses are not rituals.

They prevent escalation.

Step 4 — Fat, Carefully

Fats come later, and modestly.

This prevents:

- calorie flooding

- displacement of fat oxidation

- digestive overload

By this point, the system already accepts that food has returned.

There is no advantage to rushing.

Step 5 — Carbohydrates Only If the Day Allows

On **Wednesday**, carbohydrates are minimal or absent.
On **Saturday**, they are allowed.

But in every case, carbohydrates arrive **last**.

This prevents glucose stacking and appetite rebound.

What Happens When This Is Ignored

When a fast is broken with:

- sugar

- liquid calories

- fat-heavy foods

- fast carbohydrates

The reset does not vanish.

It **shrinks**.

Hunger returns sooner.
The next fast feels louder.
The week becomes harder than necessary.

This is not punishment.

It is physics.

The Difference Was Never the Fast

Early on, I assumed breaking the fast didn't matter.

The fast itself felt successful, so I treated re-entry casually.

The pattern was consistent:

- hunger returned the same day

- appetite felt louder

- the next fast required effort

When I slowed re-entry — acids, fibre, protein, pauses — the opposite happened.

Hunger stayed quiet.

Energy remained steady.
The next fast felt optional rather than demanding.

The fast hadn't changed.

The **re-entry had**.

Why Quiet Re-Entry Preserves the Effect

The goal of re-entry is not to end the fast.

It is to avoid undoing it.

When food returns gradually, the body remains in the same regulatory state it reached during absence. Signals stay readable. Appetite stays contained. Stored energy remains available.

When food returns abruptly, the system is forced to correct.

Insulin rises sharply.

Hunger escalates.

Eating increases.

The quiet window closes early.

Nothing has gone wrong.

The fast simply wasn't allowed to carry forward.

Quiet re-entry doesn't add discipline.

It prevents overcorrection.

It keeps the system doing what it was already doing.

The Only Line Worth Remembering

If you forget everything else in this chapter, remember this:

> **The quieter the re-entry, the longer the fast keeps working.**

Breaking a fast correctly feels uneventful.

That is how you know it worked.

CHAPTER 12 — What Actually Happens When You Tweak the Method

Real Life Doesn't Break the Method — Confusion Does

No one runs a week like this perfectly.

That was never the expectation.

What causes trouble isn't deviation.
It's **not knowing what the deviation did**.

When people believe they've "ruined everything," they overcorrect.
When they believe nothing changed, they drift.

This chapter removes both mistakes.

There is no moral language here.
There is no encouragement or discouragement.

Only **cause and effect**.

The One Principle That Governs All Deviations

The method works because it creates **long, uninterrupted periods of low insulin and low appetite signalling**.

Any deviation does one or more of the following:

- shortens that window

- raises insulin earlier than planned

- reactivates appetite signalling sooner

That's it.

Nothing explodes.
Nothing resets to zero.
Nothing is permanent.

But the cost is real, measurable, and predictable.

Eating the Evening Before a Fast

This usually happens on **Sunday night** or **Wednesday night**.

What changes

Late eating — especially sugar, starch, or fried food — keeps insulin elevated into the next morning.

As a result:

- glycogen depletion is delayed

- fat oxidation ramps later

- hunger arrives earlier

- the fast feels present instead of quiet

The fast still works.

It just works **less deeply**.

When this trade-off makes sense

- unavoidable social events

- family obligations

- one-off celebrations

This is not a mistake.
It is a choice.

How to reduce the cost

- acid before the meal

- fibre first

- protein before fat

- carbohydrates last

- stop eating earlier rather than later

You are not ruining the week.

You are shortening the runway.

Breaking a Fast Early

Sometimes a fast ends early because:

- stress spikes

- output is required

- sleep was poor

- energy drops unexpectedly

What actually happens

Breaking early:

- interrupts insulin suppression

- reduces appetite quieting

- shortens the reset

What it **does not** do is erase fat loss already achieved.

The real cost

- the next fast may feel louder

- hunger may return sooner

That's the full extent.

How to preserve most of the benefit

- re-enter with acid → fibre → protein

- avoid sugar and fat-heavy foods

- treat the break as controlled re-entry, not relief

The system responds to **how** you break, not that you broke.

Adding Carbohydrates on Sunday or Wednesday

This is usually unintentional.

What happens metabolically

Carbohydrates on these days:

- raise insulin

- restart appetite cycling

- increase hunger later that day or the next

Speed determines severity.

Why order matters more than food choice

When carbs arrive:

- after fibre

- after protein

- late in the meal

The effect is muted.

When they arrive first, they dominate the day.

The takeaway

Carbohydrates are not forbidden.

But on Sunday and Wednesday, they **set hunger tone**, not calorie load.

Fat-Loading on Wednesday

This is the most common quiet failure.

What happens

Excess dietary fat:

- replaces body-fat use

- lowers fat oxidation

- blunts the depth of the reset

Ketones may remain high — which is misleading — but fat loss slows.

Why it happens

- "It's keto, so fat is fine"

- appetite is quiet

- comfort eating returns subtly

The cost

Thursday and Friday still work —
but they have to work **harder**.

This is inefficiency, not collapse.

Moving Fast Days Around

Rearranging fast days feels harmless.

It isn't.

What changes

- hunger becomes unpredictable

- appetite probes return

- rhythm dissolves

The body prefers **predictable absence**, not creative scheduling.

When movement is acceptable

- travel

- major life events

- genuinely abnormal weeks

Frequent rearrangement removes the very thing that makes the system easy.

When Saturday Leaks Into Sunday

This is the most common long-term drift.

What happens

When Saturday extends:

- insulin stays elevated

- glycogen refills

- Monday feels louder

- hunger carries into the week

Why Sunday exists

Sunday is not punishment.

It is **repositioning**.

Returning to fibre-first, acid-primed, protein-led eating on Sunday resets the week without force.

Author Observation — What Drift Actually Felt Like

When I treated deviations casually, nothing broke immediately.

The system just got louder.

Hunger crept back in.
Fasts required effort again.
Food regained urgency.

When I restored the fixed structure — especially Sunday positioning and restrained Wednesday eating — the quiet returned without effort.

The lesson wasn't rigidity.

It was **respecting the rhythm**.

The Adult Truth

You can bend this system.

You just can't pretend it didn't bend.

Every deviation has a cost —

but the cost is temporary, predictable, and survivable.

The system does not punish.

It responds.

The Only Question That Matters After Any Deviation

Not:

"Did I mess up?"

But:

"What signal did I just reintroduce?"

Once you answer that, the next adjustment is obvious.

CHAPTER 13 — When the System No Longer Needs Pressure

The weekly eating-pause rhythm introduced earlier exists for a reason.

It clears noise.
It restores quiet signals.
It demonstrates — experientially — that hunger is mechanical rather than moral.

But it is not meant to be permanent.

Once signals are stable, continuing to apply the same level of absence does not deepen the benefit. It simply adds pressure where none is needed.

The goal of this system was never to fast regularly.
It was to remove the need for constant management.

What "Finished" Actually Looks Like

Completion does not announce itself.

There is no final fast.
No decisive number.
No moment where effort suddenly feels impressive.

Instead, the signs are behavioural:

- hunger arrives later and fades easily
- missing a meal feels neutral
- appetite does not escalate after eating

• food decisions feel boring rather than tense
• weight fluctuates within a narrow band without effort

These changes usually appear before weight loss is fully complete.

That order matters.

Stability comes first.
Weight follows quietly.

If you continue pushing after these signals are present, you are no longer resolving anything. You are applying stress to a system that has already adapted.

Why More Fasting Stops Helping

Once insulin reliably falls between meals and appetite signalling is quiet, additional fasting produces diminishing returns.

At that point:

• fat oxidation is already active
• hunger suppression is already maximal
• metabolic flexibility has been restored

What increases instead is load.

This often appears as:

• increased cold sensitivity
• lighter or disrupted sleep
• stalled progress despite consistency
• food returning to mental space

These are not failures.
They are indicators that the system no longer needs force.

What Maintenance Actually Requires

Long-term metabolic stability does not require regular extended fasting.

For most people, it comes from:

• eating in a calm sequence
• leading with fibre and protein
• avoiding stacked sugars
• allowing digestion to complete
• maintaining naturally quieter days through lighter intake

This is sufficient.

When the body trusts the environment, it stops defending.

The Role of Occasional Fasting After Stability

Some people choose to reintroduce a longer eating pause periodically — not to accelerate fat loss, but to revisit a quiet metabolic state they already recognise.

Used this way, an extended fast is not corrective.
It is optional upkeep.

This might look like:

• a single 36–48 hour pause every few weeks
• one structured week every few months
• or a brief return to the weekly rhythm during periods of drift

There is no required frequency.

If eating remains calm and signals stay quiet, more fasting adds little.
If noise returns, a short, deliberate reset often resolves it quickly.

The difference is intent.

This is not pressure.
It is maintenance.

Stepping Back Without Losing Stability

Reducing fasting does not mean abandoning structure.

What stays:

• sequencing
• pacing
• delayed dessert
• unstacked carbohydrates

What changes is how often absence is used.

Removing pressure while preserving order is not regression.
It is graduation.

If signals worsen, the feedback is immediate.
If they remain quiet, nothing needs fixing.

The Only Principle That Endures

Fasting was never the goal.

It was the fastest way to show you that hunger was never the enemy — and that stability does not require control.

Once that lesson is embodied, the system sustains itself.

Nothing here is fragile.

That is the point.

CHAPTER 14 — Refinements, Not Rules

When (and Why) to Add Variations

By this point, the system should feel familiar.

Meals are paced.
Weeks have rhythm.
Signals are readable instead of chaotic.

That's the foundation.

Everything in this chapter sits **on top of that foundation**, not in place of it.

Refinements are not necessary to make the method work. Many people never need them. Weight stabilises. Appetite stays calm. Life fits.

So before anything else, it's important to be clear about intent.

You don't add variations because something is wrong.
You add them because the structure is already stable.

Refinements exist for three reasons only:

- to accommodate changing circumstances

- to reduce friction in specific situations

- to support the rhythm during periods of stress, travel, or transition

They are not accelerators.

Trying to use refinements to force faster results usually backfires. It reintroduces decision-making and complexity — the very things the core method removed.

This chapter is about **optional tools**, not progress gates.

Some people will reach a point where their routine changes.

Work schedules shift.
Travel increases.
Social eating becomes more frequent.
Physical demands rise.

In those cases, small adjustments can help the rhythm hold without requiring more effort.

Others may notice that appetite has stabilised enough that quieter days feel almost automatic — and they're curious whether gentle variations still preserve calm.

That curiosity is healthy.

What matters is that refinements are introduced **one at a time**, with observation — not stacked all at once.

The system works best when cause and effect remain clear.

If something improves stability, it earns a place.
If it adds effort without benefit, it's removed.

There is no hierarchy here.

Using more tools does not mean you're doing the method better.
In many cases, the opposite is true.

The simplest version that holds is the best version.

The sections that follow will introduce a handful of refinements that people commonly find useful once the rhythm is established.

Each one stands alone.
None are required.
All are reversible.

Think of them as ways to *support* stability — not ways to replace it.

Using Refinements to Reduce Friction, Not Add Effort

The most useful refinements do not change the structure of the method.

They remove friction around it.

Friction is anything that makes the rhythm harder to maintain than it needs to be — not because the method is flawed, but because life introduces constraints the default shape wasn't designed to anticipate.

Long workdays.
Irregular schedules.
Travel.
Social obligations that cluster unpredictably.

In these situations, the mistake is trying to force the default week to fit perfectly.

Refinements exist to absorb pressure without breaking contrast.

The first principle to keep in mind is this:

A refinement should **make the rhythm easier to hold**, not more impressive to execute.

If a variation adds planning, tracking, or vigilance, it's probably unnecessary.

A good refinement has three characteristics:

- it preserves clear contrast across the week

- it reduces decision-making in specific situations

- it can be removed without destabilising anything

One common example is **adjusting where quieter days sit**, without changing their role.

Some weeks make it obvious that spacing quieter days differently would reduce stress. Placing them closer together, or anchoring them to predictable low-demand days, often makes them calmer rather than harder.

This isn't an optimisation.

It's alignment.

Another example is **simplifying eating days when life is busy.**

Instead of trying to maintain variety or novelty, eating days can become deliberately repetitive for a period. Familiar meals reduce decision load, shorten negotiation, and help appetite remain settled when attention is pulled elsewhere.

Nothing about the method requires novelty.

Stability often improves when complexity drops.

A third example is **supporting quieter days during high stress**.

Stress amplifies hunger signals. In those periods, refinements might involve reducing friction around hydration, sleep, or workload — not altering food structure itself.

The key is recognising what problem you're solving.

If the problem is "this feels harder than it should," a refinement may help.
If the problem is "I want faster results," a refinement is unlikely to help.

Refinements should always be introduced with observation.

Try one change.
Watch how appetite responds across several days.
Keep what genuinely reduces effort.

If nothing improves, revert.

There is no penalty for simplicity.

In the next section, we'll look at refinements specific to **social and travel contexts** — situations where rigidity fails quickly, and where small adjustments can preserve rhythm without drawing attention or requiring explanation.

When Life Gets Social, Mobile, or Unpredictable

Most methods break down in social situations.

Not because the food is different, but because the context is.

Meals stretch longer.
Choices are limited or shared.
Timing is out of your control.
Attention is on people, not structure.

This is where rigidity fails.

The goal in these situations is not to preserve the *form* of the method, but its **function**.

That function is simple:
keep contrast across the week, and keep meals from accelerating unnecessarily.

Everything else is optional.

In social settings, the most useful refinement is **selective attention**.

You don't need to manage the entire meal. You only need to be aware of how it begins. Letting the opening slow down — even briefly — often does enough work that the rest of the meal takes care of itself.

You're not eating differently from anyone else.
You're just not rushing the fastest parts to the front.

Once the pace is set, the situation usually stabilises.

Travel presents a different challenge.

Schedules compress. Food availability narrows. Eating becomes opportunistic rather than planned.

Here, the mistake is trying to recreate ideal conditions.

Instead, focus on **preserving roles**, not timing.

An eating day is still an eating day, even if meals are simpler or less varied. A quieter day is still a quieter day, even if it looks different from home.

What matters is that the distinction remains clear.

If travel collapses everything into constant grazing, appetite becomes reactive quickly. If contrast is maintained — even imperfectly — the system holds far better than expected.

Another useful refinement in these contexts is **lowering expectations, not standards**.

You're not aiming for optimal meals.
You're aiming for meals that don't create instability.

That often means accepting repetition, simplicity, or less-than-ideal choices — without compensating later.

Compensation is what breaks rhythm.

If a social meal is larger or richer than usual, the response is not restriction. It's allowing the next quieter day to do its job without interference.

If travel disrupts a quieter day, the response is not doubling up later. It's restoring contrast when circumstances allow.

The method survives these contexts because it doesn't require explanation.

You don't need to announce anything.
You don't need to decline participation.

You don't need to justify choices.

You're not "on" something.

You're simply maintaining a rhythm that adapts to where you are.

In the next section, we'll look at refinements that support **high physical demand** — periods of training, labour, or increased activity — and how to accommodate them without reintroducing instability.

Supporting High Activity Without Losing Stability

There will be periods when your physical demands increase.

Training intensifies.
Work becomes more manual.
Daily movement rises sharply.

In these moments, appetite often changes — sometimes dramatically.

The common mistake is assuming that higher activity requires abandoning structure. People shift into constant fueling, frequent eating, or unstructured compensation. Hunger gets louder. The rhythm dissolves.

That response is understandable.

It's also unnecessary.

Higher activity doesn't change the core principle of the method.

It changes **how much support eating days need**, not whether rhythm applies.

The first thing to understand is this:

Increased output does not require constant input.

The body is well equipped to mobilise energy when signals are clear. What disrupts that process is not demand — it's instability.

When activity rises, the system needs two things:

- eating days that are genuinely complete

- quieter days that still create space, even if they look different

Eating days may need to carry more load.

That doesn't mean grazing all day.
It means allowing meals to be fully satisfying so recovery can occur.

Cutting eating days short during high activity is one of the fastest ways to destabilise appetite. Hunger sharpens, cravings escalate, and the week becomes reactive.

Quieter days may need adjustment as well.

They may not be as minimal as during lower-demand periods — and that's fine. What matters is that they remain **distinct**. Reduced intake, simplified structure, and clear spacing still allow signals to settle even when output is high.

The error is turning every day into a partial eating day.

That blurs contrast and keeps the system busy.

Another important refinement during high activity is **respecting recovery signals**.

Sleep disruption, lingering soreness, or unusual fatigue often indicate that the system is under load. In those cases, the rhythm should support recovery, not push through it.

This might mean temporarily prioritising eating-day completeness over strict contrast. Or spacing quieter days differently so they don't coincide with peak demand.

None of this is optimisation.

It's preservation.

The method isn't designed to compete with training cycles or labour schedules. It's designed to adapt to them without losing stability.

If activity increases and appetite stays calm, the structure is working.

If activity increases and appetite becomes chaotic, the solution is almost always to **restore clarity** — clearer eating days, clearer quieter days, fewer interruptions in between.

The principle doesn't change.

Only the load does.

In the next section, we'll step back and look at how to decide whether a refinement is actually helping — and when the best move is to remove it and return to the simplest version of the rhythm.

Knowing When to Remove a Refinement

Refinements are meant to support stability — not replace it.

Over time, it's easy for small adjustments to accumulate. A tweak for travel stays in place afterward. A variation for stress becomes habitual. What started as support quietly turns into structure.

That's when effort creeps back in.

The simplest test for any refinement is this:

Does this make the rhythm easier to hold — or harder to think about?

If a variation reduces decision-making, lowers friction, and keeps appetite calm, it earns its place.

If it requires monitoring, planning, or explanation, it probably doesn't.

Most refinements are situational. They solve a specific problem for a specific period. Once that period passes, the refinement should pass with it.

Keeping it "just in case" often adds more load than benefit.

There is no advantage to complexity here.

Using more tools does not deepen the method. In most cases, it dilutes it.

The core rhythm is intentionally minimal because minimal systems recover faster. When something drifts, it's easier to see.

When life changes, it's easier to adapt.

This is why returning to the simplest version is always a valid move.

If appetite becomes noisy, simplify.
If the week feels heavy, simplify.
If eating starts occupying mental space again, simplify.

Removing refinements is not regression.

It's recalibration.

Many people find that after a period of experimentation, they naturally settle back into a stripped-down rhythm — one or two eating days doing their job well, one or two quieter days creating space, and the rest of the week unfolding without much thought.

That's not settling for less.

That's arriving.

This chapter isn't about building a personalised system you have to manage.

It's about discovering how little structure is actually required once stability returns.

In the next chapter, we'll step out of refinement entirely and address a different concern: how to live inside this rhythm long-term without it becoming an identity or something you feel you have to protect.

CHAPTER 15 — Living With the Rhythm

When the Method Disappears

At some point, something subtle happens.

You stop thinking about the method.

Days pass without reference to structure. Meals happen without analysis. The week unfolds without negotiation.

That isn't a loss of discipline.

It's the outcome.

Most systems fail quietly by becoming identities. People don't just follow them — they explain them, protect them, and feel threatened when life challenges them.

This method was never meant to live in the foreground.

If it does, something has gone wrong.

The rhythm exists to stabilise appetite, not to occupy attention. Once stability holds, it should recede.

You don't wake up thinking about contrast.
You don't evaluate every meal.
You don't feel the need to "stay on track."

The track is already underneath you.

That's why the structure avoids rigid rules and declarations. Anything that requires defence eventually becomes fragile.

A rhythm that works is quiet.

It tolerates holidays.
It tolerates stress.
It tolerates seasons of change.

Living with the rhythm long-term means letting it become
context, not content.

You notice drift without alarm.
You restore contrast without drama.
You simplify when weeks get noisy.

There's no sense of starting or stopping.

Food is no longer something you manage.

It's simply no longer chaotic.

How This Holds Across Time — Even When Old Fears Return

No rhythm stays static.

Life changes.
Bodies change.
Priorities shift.

What makes this approach durable is that it adapts **without needing redesign**.

The roles stay the same, even as their expression softens or
sharpens.

During calm periods, contrast emerges naturally. Appetite settles quickly. Food fades further into the background.

During demanding periods — illness, travel, stress, grief — the rhythm flexes. Quieter days may shorten. Eating days may simplify rather than complete.

That isn't failure.

It's responsiveness.

Over time, many people notice something else as well: old fears resurface occasionally.

A small weight change.
A comment from someone else.
A familiar thought — *What if this stops working?*

These moments aren't warnings.

They're memory.

Most people didn't arrive here casually. The nervous system remembers years of vigilance and effort. When uncertainty appears, the impulse to control can return quickly.

This is the critical point.

Not because something needs fixing — but because acting on fear is how the old cycle restarts.

Stability wasn't created through urgency.
It was created through consistency.

When fear appears, the most effective response isn't reassurance. It's orientation.

What is actually happening right now?
Has the rhythm broken — or just softened?
Is life under unusual load?

Most of the time, nothing fundamental has changed.

Fear often passes when it isn't immediately corrected — just like
hunger did earlier in the process.

Each time you allow the structure to hold without interference,
trust deepens.

Eventually, fear visits less often.
When it does, it carries less authority.
And when it leaves, you barely notice.

That isn't discipline.

It's safety returning.

What This Actually Gives You Back

By now, it should be clear that this was never just about weight.

Weight changes were the visible effect — not the core repair.

What this method restores is something quieter, and far more
valuable.

It gives you back **neutrality**.

Food loses emotional charge.
Hunger stops feeling threatening.
Eating no longer requires explanation — to yourself or anyone
else.

That neutrality is what most people have been chasing without realising it.

Not control.
Not perfection.
But the absence of constant management.

When the system stabilises, effort falls away in places you didn't expect.

You think ahead less.
You review meals less.
You stop bracing for consequences.

Food becomes part of life again, not a variable you're constantly adjusting.

Weight follows the same pattern.

It stops feeling precarious.
It stops feeling like something that could unravel if you relax.
It stops occupying mental space.

That doesn't mean nothing ever changes.

It means change no longer feels dangerous.

You trust that if something drifts, it can settle again — because you've watched it happen. Repeatedly. Through busy weeks, stress, social periods, and quiet stretches.

That trust isn't optimism.

It's evidence.

This is why the method doesn't end with rules or targets.

Those would imply fragility.

Instead, it ends with a capacity you now have: the ability to create stability when it's needed — and to let it fade into the background when it's not.

Most people spend years trying to override their appetite.

This approach teaches you how to stop provoking it.

Once that happens, the struggle dissolves on its own.

You don't become disciplined.

You become **unbothered**.

And that — more than any number on a scale — is what makes the change permanent.

CHAPTER 16 — Living Inside the System

How This Becomes Normal Life (Without Vigilance)

By the time most people reach this point, something important has already happened.

The method has stopped feeling like a method.

Meals are quieter.
Hunger is predictable.
Eating decisions no longer feel loaded.

That change is not accidental — and it is not fragile.

This chapter explains how the system settles into daily life, why it holds without constant attention, and what "normal" looks like once the work of Part 2 is finished.

The Moment the System Stops Being Active

There is a distinct shift that occurs after a few cycles of the Accelerator.

You stop asking:

- "Is this allowed?"

- "Should I eat now?"

- "Am I doing this right?"

And start noticing:

- hunger arrives later

- smaller meals satisfy

- skipping food feels neutral

- eating feels procedural rather than emotional

This is the point where **control dissolves into structure.**

Not because rules were memorised — but because signals stopped colliding.

A Subtle Shift You May Notice

Around this point, many people notice another quiet change.

Portion size begins adjusting on its own — not because of restraint, but because timing has become legible. Meals start to resolve earlier. Satisfaction arrives sooner. Eating past that point feels neutral rather than compelling.

What's less obvious — until it happens a few times — is how this begins to coordinate with life outside the meal itself.

If there is a social dinner later, a shared event, or a known eating window ahead, earlier meals often end smaller without planning. Not skipped. Not reduced deliberately. Simply finished sooner. The body no longer behaves as if it must carry excess forward "just in case."

This is not foresight. It's trust.

When appetite is no longer defending against unpredictable intake, it stops overshooting. Meals end where they should, because the system no longer needs insurance. Food doesn't have to last until the next opportunity — it will arrive when expected.

Most people only notice this in hindsight:
"I wasn't especially full — I just didn't need more."
"I stopped earlier than usual and didn't think about it again."
"I ate less because there was something later — without trying to."

This is not discipline.
It is signal resolution extending beyond the plate.

You may also notice a new choice becoming available.

Meals can be sized with an end in mind — not to restrict intake, but to align with what comes next. When another eating context is expected later, the meal can be allowed to close earlier. When the day is quiet, it can be allowed to finish fully.

The decision is no longer "How much should I eat?"
It becomes "How long does this meal need to carry me?"

This is not optimisation.
It is coordination.

Because signals are stable, choosing to stop earlier does not create anxiety or rebound. Appetite understands timing. It no longer demands excess to protect against uncertainty.

This is one of the clearest signs the system is working.
Not because you are trying to eat less — but because you can choose when a meal is complete, and trust that choice.

When eating becomes predictable, portions become contextual.

And when portions become contextual, effort quietly disappears.

What Actually Holds the Weight Off

Long-term stability in this system does not come from fasting.

It comes from **three structural habits** that remain even when fasting fades:

1. **Order**
   - fibre first
   - protein before energy
   - carbs last
   - dessert delayed or substituted

2. **Speed**
   - food enters slowly
   - digestion is not rushed
   - signals have time to register

3. **Boundaries**
   - indulgence is bounded in time
   - sugar is contextual, not ambient
   - eating does not spill across days

These do not require effort once they are familiar.

They replace vigilance with default behaviour.

What Normal Eating Looks Like Now

Normal eating in this system does not look "clean."

It looks **uninteresting**.

Meals are assembled without drama.
Foods repeat.
Decisions are simple.

You may still eat:

- carbohydrates

- desserts

- fried foods

- social meals

But they occur:

- after structure

- within time bounds

- without compensation afterward

The absence of guilt is not discipline.

It is **predictability**.

Why Appetite No Longer Escalates

Earlier in the book, you learned that appetite escalates when:

- food arrives too fast

- sugar stacks

- insulin cycles repeatedly

- reward is unbounded

By this stage, those conditions rarely occur together.

Even when one appears, the others usually do not.

That is why appetite no longer "runs away."

The system does not rely on suppression.

It relies on **preventing convergence**.

The Quiet Skill You Now Have

Most people believe appetite control is about restraint.

What you now have instead is **timing literacy**.

You can feel when:

- hunger is mechanical

- hunger is anticipatory

- hunger is reward-driven

- hunger is stress-driven

And because you can identify it, you can respond without urgency.

This is not willpower.

It is pattern recognition.

What Happens When Life Gets Chaotic

Travel, illness, stress, and disruption still happen.

When they do, one of two things occurs:

- either the system dampens the impact automatically

- or appetite noise returns briefly and predictably

The key difference now is that nothing is mysterious.

You don't spiral.
You don't "start over."
You simply reintroduce the missing structure.

Usually:

- fibre-first meals

- delayed sugar

- one low-insulin day

That is enough.

When I Stopped Monitoring Altogether

The point where I knew the system had integrated was when I stopped checking anything.

No tracking.
No timing obsession.
No rules running in the background.

Eating happened.

Weight stayed stable.

Hunger stayed quiet.

When I later reintroduced the Accelerator intentionally, it felt like a tool — not a requirement.

That distinction matters.

The Difference Between a Method and an Operating System

A method is something you apply.

An operating system is something you live inside.

The Artisan Method stops being something you "do" once:

- hunger becomes predictable

- eating loses urgency

- weight stabilises without negotiation

From that point on, fasting is optional.

Structure is not.

Where This Leaves You

You are no longer dependent on:

- perfect weeks

- strict plans

- constant restraint

You understand:

- what signals matter
- how to quiet them
- how to restore order when needed

Nothing here requires belief.

Everything here is repeatable.

Closing the Arc

The goal of this project was never to make you better at resisting food.

It was to make **resistance unnecessary**.

Once that happens, the rest of life fits back in — without effort.

CHAPTER 17 — Nothing to Defend

Why This Lasts Without Belief

By the end of this book, something subtle should be true.

You are not trying to remember rules.
You are not holding a plan together.
You are not protecting progress from collapse.

There is nothing to defend.

That absence is the outcome.

Most approaches to weight loss end by asking you to *maintain* something.
Maintenance implies vigilance.
Vigilance implies threat.

This system was designed so that nothing fragile is ever created in the first place.

Why This Does Not Require Faith

Nothing you've read asks you to believe a theory.

Everything asks you to notice a response.

- Eat fibre first and hunger softens.

- Delay sugar and appetite does not escalate.

- Remove insulin cycling and fat loss resumes.

- Fast when signals are quiet and effort disappears.

These are not ideas.

They are **observations you can repeat**.

That repeatability is why the system holds without belief.

The Shift Most People Miss

The biggest mistake people make at the end of a successful intervention is trying to *preserve the intervention.*

They keep fasting because it worked.
They keep restricting because it produced change.
They keep controlling because they fear reversal.

That fear is what reintroduces instability.

The Artisan Method works because it **removes the need for defence**.

Once hunger is quiet and eating is ordered, weight stabilises by default.

Nothing needs protecting.

Why Regain Is Not a Mystery Anymore

If weight ever drifts again, you will know why.

Not abstractly.
Mechanically.

You will recognise whether:

- sugar became ambient

- meals sped up

- fibre disappeared

- reward leaked across days

- insulin lost its low baseline

There is no panic in that recognition.

There is only a clear lever to pull.

That clarity is the real safeguard.

What Success Actually Feels Like

Success here does not feel victorious.

It feels dull.

Food loses narrative weight.
Eating loses emotional charge.
Body weight becomes a background metric rather than a project.

If you are waiting for pride or excitement, you may miss it.

The signal that this worked is **indifference**.

The Moment I Knew the Problem Was Gone

The moment this stopped being a "system" for me was when I forgot it for weeks.

Not because I was avoiding it — but because nothing required attention.

When stress hit, eating did not escalate.
When routine broke, hunger did not spike.
When structure returned, everything settled without effort.

That is when I realised the problem had been solved, not managed.

Why This Is Not a Lifestyle Brand

There are no communities to join.
No products to buy.
No identities to adopt.

Those things create dependency.

This book exists to **remove dependency** — including on the book itself.

Once you understand the mechanics, the text becomes unnecessary.

That is intentional.

The Only Thing to Carry Forward

If you carry one thing with you, let it be this:

> Hunger is not a character flaw.
> Weight is not a moral outcome.
> Appetite responds to structure, speed, and sequence — nothing else.

When those are in place, the body cooperates.

When they are not, it resists.

That is not failure.

It is feedback.

Closing the Loop

You do not need to start again.
You do not need to optimise further.
You do not need to push harder.

If something drifts, you already know what to restore.

That is enough.

Nothing here depends on perfection.
Nothing here requires defence.

The system works because it **lets go**.

CHAPTER 18 — Common Questions and Clarifications

This chapter exists to answer questions that tend to arise once people begin applying the method in real life.

They are not prerequisites.
They are not rules.
They are not exceptions that need to be memorised.

Most readers will not need every entry here. Many will not need any of them at all.

But when eating patterns begin to change, certain situations predictably surface:
busy days, shared meals, unexpected hunger, social pressure, stalled progress, or advice that seems to contradict what you are observing.

Rather than addressing these throughout the main text, they are collected here so the core method can remain clean and uninterrupted.

Each section responds to a common point of friction—not by adding control, but by returning to first principles:
pace, sequence, and rhythm.

If something in your day feels unclear, unsettled, or louder than expected, this chapter is a place to check alignment before assuming something is wrong.

Read selectively.
Use what applies.

Ignore what doesn't.

If a situation resolves appetite, steadies energy, and reduces noise, it is working—whether or not it appears here.

The material that follows is not a second method layered on top of the first.
It is the same method, viewed from angles people often ask about once they start living with it.

How to Open a Meal When Life Is Busy

These examples are not templates. They're illustrations of how pacing shows up naturally when life isn't tidy.

Most meals don't fail because of what's on the plate.

They unravel because everything arrives too fast.

When life is busy, the idea of "doing meals properly" can feel unrealistic. There isn't time to plan openings, prepare starters, or sit everyone down at once. That's fine. The body doesn't need perfection. It needs **a moment to set the pace**.

Even a small delay at the beginning of a meal changes how digestion unfolds.

That delay doesn't have to look special.

It can be a bowl of vegetables already in the fridge.
A simple salad with oil and acid.
A cup of yoghurt without sugar.
A mug of soup, tea, or something warm while food finishes cooking.

180

None of these are "rules." They're ways of buying time.

When the first thing the body receives takes a little longer to break down, digestion starts more slowly. Signals rise in an orderly way. The rest of the meal enters a system that's already working — instead of forcing it to accelerate all at once.

This is why openings matter more than ingredients.

A perfect meal eaten quickly behaves like a fast one. An imperfect meal that starts slowly often holds.

On busy days, the most effective change is often the smallest: **don't let the meal begin at full speed**.

If you can create even a few minutes between hunger and dense energy arriving, the system responds. Appetite settles earlier. Urgency softens. Eating feels quieter without trying to make it so.

Over time, this becomes automatic.

You stop thinking about "opening a meal" and start noticing when meals feel different. The ones that hold. The ones that don't ask for follow-up. The ones that let food fade into the background again.

The structure does the work.

Your job is just to give it a moment to start.

Family Meals Without Turning Dinner Into a Project

Family meals rarely unfold calmly on their own.

Someone is hungry early.
Someone else is distracted.
The food isn't ready at the same time for everyone.

Trying to force order onto that usually backfires.

What works better is letting the meal **unfold in stages**, without announcing that you're doing anything differently.

A common scene looks like this.

The kids are hungry and hovering while dinner is still fifteen minutes away. Instead of rushing the main or asking them to wait, something simple comes out first — a small salad with oil and acid, a bowl of vegetables already prepared, a chia–yoghurt cup without sugar, or a mug of soup or tea.

Nothing heavy. Nothing dramatic.

While they eat that, the vegetables finish cooking. Adjustments are made to the main. The sense of urgency drops.

If someone gets up, wanders off, or fidgets, that's fine. Movement between courses isn't a problem — it actually creates space for each stage of the meal to settle before the next arrives.

When the vegetables are ready, they're served.
"The rest isn't quite ready yet."

By the time protein and fats come to the table, hunger has changed character. Eating slows on its own. Carbohydrates — especially baked or fried ones — arrive last, once people are already eating instead of waiting.

Nothing about this is framed as a rule.

There's no talk of "order" or "structure."
The meal just stretches instead of compressing.

Later, instead of dessert appearing immediately, the table clears. Homework starts. The dog gets walked. A movie is picked. An hour passes.

Sometimes dessert still happens. Sometimes it doesn't. Popcorn with butter and salt often feels like enough. The point isn't avoidance — it's **delay**.

What makes this work is that no one is being managed.

The pauses are built into normal family flow: cooking, clearing, moving, transitioning. Each stage gives the body time to process what arrived before the next thing shows up.

One important note about the table itself.

Shared meals work best when the table stays emotionally quiet. Asking about the day is fine. Listening is better. Offering advice — even well-intentioned — often makes sitting together tense.

If something comes up that needs guidance, it's better handled later: on the couch, in a bedroom, or while walking the dog. The table should build closeness, not become a place where people brace themselves.

That matters more than it sounds.

When meals feel safe and unpressured, digestion settles more easily. The method holds. Family time improves. Eating becomes something everyone moves through — not something they have to endure.

The structure isn't strict.

It's simply patient enough to let everyone arrive.

Eating Out, Shared Plates, and Social Meals

Most eating happens away from ideal conditions.

Meals are shared.
Orders arrive out of sequence.
You don't control what's on the table — or when.

That doesn't make pacing irrelevant. It just changes how quietly it's applied.

When you're eating out, the simplest move is to let **something slow arrive first**, even if it's small. A vegetable side. A starter. Soup. Anything that asks the system to begin working before dense energy shows up.

If nothing like that is available, time itself can do the job.

Let others start first.
Take a few minutes before eating.
Sip a drink. Talk. Settle.

That pause matters more than it looks like it should.

With shared plates, the same principle applies. You don't need to avoid anything. You don't need to control the order for the table. You only need to notice what you reach for first.

If faster foods are already moving around, let them arrive **into** an already active system instead of being the opening act. A few bites later behaves very differently than the same food eaten immediately.

This is why social meals often feel better when you're not the first one eating.

The pace has already been set.

Nothing here requires explanation or negotiation. You're not "doing" the method in public. You're simply allowing the meal to unfold instead of rushing to fill the first gap.

That's also why this works at events.

Finger food. Buffets. Grazing tables.

You don't need to track or restrict. You only need to delay the first dense input long enough for digestion to begin at a manageable speed.

Once eating is in motion, the system is far more tolerant. Foods that would have caused urgency on an empty stomach often pass through quietly when they arrive later.

Social meals don't need to be optimised.

They just need to start slowly enough for the body to keep up.

When that happens, you leave feeling connected — not depleted or overcorrecting later.

The structure stays invisible.

That's how it's meant to work.

Breakfast: Essential, Optional, or Conditional?

Many dietary guidelines emphasise the importance of breakfast. This advice exists for a reason — but it is often misunderstood.

At a population level, skipping breakfast is associated with overeating later in the day, unstable energy, and poorer food choices. In environments shaped by long workdays, stress, and ultra-processed food, eating early often reduces harm.

The Artisan Method approaches the same question from a different angle.

What matters is not the clock.
It is the state of the system when the first food arrives.

Some people wake hungry. Others do not. In many cases, the absence of morning hunger reflects unfinished digestion or correction from the previous day, not a lack of fuel. Adding fast energy at that point often creates the mid-morning crashes people are trying to avoid.

This does not mean breakfast should be skipped.
It means breakfast is conditional.

The method does not ask whether you eat in the morning.
It asks whether the day opens calmly or under correction.

A sugar-dominant or rushed opening tends to accelerate

digestion before the system has stabilised. A slower opening — or a later first meal once hunger is clear — allows signals to settle before energy ramps up. Both approaches can work. The difference is pace.

The examples below are not recommendations. They illustrate how the same principle adapts to different mornings.

Some people find that eating early helps the day stay steady. In that case, a calm opening is usually small, slow, and unspectacular. It begins without sweetness or urgency. The goal is not to feel energised, but to prevent the day from accelerating before it needs to.

Others notice that they are not hungry until mid-morning. When access to food later is predictable, waiting often allows overnight processes to finish cleanly. Hunger arrives more clearly, and the first meal is easier to pace. In this case, delaying the opening creates less correction than forcing one.

When the day will be constrained by travel or long gaps, eating before leaving can be stabilising even without hunger. The purpose is not to "fuel up," but to set a manageable pace before options narrow. A slow opening early is usually quieter than a rushed one later.

The Artisan Method does not treat breakfast as a rule to follow or a habit to break. It treats it as an opening — one that sets the speed for everything that follows.

Dessert Without Undoing the Meal

Dessert rarely causes problems because of what it is.

It causes problems because of **when** it arrives.

When something sweet or fast appears immediately after a meal, it often lands while digestion is still accelerating. The system hasn't finished processing what came before, so the additional energy stacks on top of an already rising curve.

That's when things unravel.

What changes the outcome isn't avoidance — it's **delay**.

When there's a pause after eating, the body gets time to finish its work. Signals settle. Appetite softens. By the time dessert is considered, the urgency that drove it earlier has often passed.

In practice, this pause usually looks like transition.

The table is cleared.
Dishes are done.
Homework starts.
A walk happens.
A movie is chosen.

An hour is often enough.

Sometimes dessert still fits. Sometimes it doesn't. What's different is that it arrives as a choice, not a reflex.

This is why dessert feels completely different during a movie than it does at the table. Eating later happens against a calmer background. The system isn't scrambling to catch up.

Popcorn with butter and salt often works well here — not because it's virtuous, but because it arrives slowly and is eaten slowly. Sugar-heavy desserts tend to do the opposite.

The goal isn't to eliminate treats.

It's to stop them from **restarting digestion at full speed**.

Over time, something else happens.

When meals finish cleanly, dessert often loses its pull. Not because you're resisting it — but because the system doesn't ask for it as loudly.

That's the signal you're looking for.

Not restraint.
Completion.

When digestion finishes its work, appetite usually moves on with it.

Dessert becomes optional — and that's when it fits best.

Headaches, Fatigue, and When Something Feels Wrong

On quieter days, discomfort doesn't always show up as hunger.

Sometimes it shows up as a dull headache.
A flat, irritable feeling.
Lightheadedness when standing.
Cold hands or feet.

A sense that energy is missing, even though you're not tired in the usual way.

These sensations are easy to misread.

They're often labelled as low energy, lack of will, or a sign that the day is "too hard." In reality, they usually have nothing to do with effort.

They're signs of **depletion**, not deprivation.

When eating pauses and insulin stays low for longer stretches, the body begins releasing stored water and sodium. This is a normal response to reduced intake. It's part of how the system resets and clears unfinished signals.

But because little or no food is coming in on quieter days, that sodium isn't being replaced through meals.

Water follows sodium.

If neither is replenished, the day can feel far harder than it needs to be.

This kind of depletion doesn't improve by pushing through. It doesn't resolve with distraction. And it often doesn't respond to food in the way hunger does.

That's the clue.

When eating doesn't help — and time doesn't soften the feeling — the issue usually isn't energy. It's balance.

Hydration often needs to be more intentional on these days. Sodium may need to be replaced in simple forms that don't restart digestion.

And thirst still matters.

If you're feeling thirsty, drink.

When fluids are adequate and salt is replaced appropriately, these symptoms often resolve quickly. The day settles. Mental noise drops. Energy steadies in a way that feels surprisingly calm.

This isn't something to fight.

If a quieter day feels agitating or uncomfortable, it usually means too much is missing — not that you're doing something wrong.

The goal is quiet, not endurance.

When balance is restored, the calm returns with it.

When Hunger Feels Loud

Not all hunger means the same thing.

One of the most common reasons people abandon a new eating pattern is because hunger shows up loudly — and they assume something has gone wrong.

Often, it hasn't.

Loud hunger usually isn't a demand for immediate intake. It's a signal that **something is unfinished**.

When digestion has been interrupted repeatedly — by frequent meals, snacks, or fast openings — appetite never gets to complete its cycle. Signals rise, get cut off, then rise again. Over time, hunger becomes sharper, earlier, and harder to ignore. These patterns become easier to distinguish with repetition; early confusion is normal.

This kind of hunger has a frantic quality.
It feels urgent.
Distracting.
Insistent in a way that doesn't soften with time.

That's different from hunger that arrives after digestion has actually finished.

Finished hunger tends to come later.
It's steadier.
Easier to sit alongside normal activity.
More responsive to a simple meal.

Another source of loud hunger is habit.

Eating at the same times every day — especially with frequent reinforcement — trains appetite to expect input whether digestion is complete or not. When that expectation isn't met, hunger appears on schedule even if the body doesn't need energy yet.

There's also hunger that comes from depletion.

This one is often misread.

When sodium or fluid levels drop, the body can produce sensations that feel like hunger but don't respond to food. Eating doesn't settle them. Time doesn't help. They linger or worsen.

That's why interpretation matters.

Not all hunger should be acted on immediately.
Not all hunger should be ignored.
And not all hunger is solved by eating more.

The purpose of structure is to make these differences easier to feel.

As meals quiet down and digestion completes more often, hunger changes character. It becomes less demanding. More informative. Easier to respond to without urgency.

When hunger softens with time, it's often safe to wait.
When it sharpens despite waiting, something else is usually missing.

The goal isn't to suppress hunger.

It's to let it finish what it's trying to do.

When Weight Stalls or Fluctuates

Weight rarely changes in a straight line.

One of the most confusing moments for many people comes after things start to feel better — meals hold longer, hunger quiets, energy steadies — but the scale doesn't move, or even moves the wrong way.

That pause is often misread as failure.

In reality, it's usually **recalibration.**

When digestion slows and insulin exposure drops, the body begins shifting how it handles water, sodium, and stored fuel. These changes happen first. Fat loss follows later.

During this phase, weight can stall.
It can fluctuate up and down.
It can hide behind water shifts for weeks.

None of that means progress isn't happening.

A quieter system often stabilises before it releases.

This is why reacting too early causes problems. Tightening intake, adding restrictions, or forcing additional changes usually reintroduces noise just as the system is settling.

The scale responds to trends, not moments.

What matters more than daily numbers is whether appetite is finishing its work more often. Meals that don't demand follow-up. Days that don't require constant correction.

Those are signs that the underlying pattern is changing.

Another common source of confusion is comparison.

Two people can follow the same structure and see different timelines. Body size, history, stress, sleep, and prior dieting all affect how quickly visible change appears.

That variability isn't a flaw in the method. It's evidence that the method is **responding to real systems**, not enforcing a template.

If weight is fluctuating but hunger is quieter, stay steady.

If energy is more even and meals hold longer, stay steady.

Quiet systems change first.
Scales follow later.

Patience here isn't passive.

It's letting the body finish what it has already started.

Foods That Tend to Slow the Opening

Some foods naturally ask the body to work before energy arrives.

They take time to chew.
They take time to break down.
They occupy the digestive system long enough for signals to rise in an orderly way.

When these foods arrive first, digestion sets a calmer pace for everything that follows.

This isn't about choosing "better" foods. It's about noticing **what tends to slow the opening.**

Foods with intact structure usually do this well.

Fibrous vegetables are a common example. Leafy greens, cruciferous vegetables, and anything that still feels like a plant rather than a paste tend to move more slowly through the system.

Soups and broths can also slow the start, especially when they're warm and savoury. They introduce volume and warmth without delivering dense energy all at once.

Textured foods matter here. Foods that require chewing, cutting, or effort to eat tend to engage digestion gradually. That engagement is what sets the pace.

Protein-first foods often sit comfortably in this category as well. While protein doesn't convert quickly into usable energy, it does stimulate digestion. When it arrives into an empty system, it can help establish a measured rhythm rather than a rush.

None of these foods are magic.

They don't guarantee stability on their own.

They simply tend to **buy time**.

When the opening of a meal takes longer to move through the body, the rest of the meal is absorbed into that slower current. Faster foods that arrive later are less likely to overwhelm the system because digestion is already underway.

This is why the same meal can feel completely different depending on how it starts.

The point isn't to memorise lists.

It's to recognise the pattern.

Foods that slow the opening don't need to be perfect. They just need to arrive first often enough for the body to set a manageable speed.

Once that happens, the rest becomes easier to live with — and easier to forget about once the meal is done.

Foods That Tend to Accelerate Digestion

Some foods move through the body very quickly.

They break down easily.
They convert rapidly.
They deliver usable energy before digestion has had time to settle.

When these foods arrive early in a meal, they often set a pace the rest of the meal can't slow down.

This doesn't make them "bad."

It means they are **fast**.

Refined starches are the most obvious example. Foods that have been ground, flaked, puffed, or softened tend to present a large surface area to digestion. Energy becomes available almost immediately.

Sugar does this even more directly. When sugar arrives early — especially without fibre or structure — signals rise sharply and corrections begin right away.

Combinations of sugar and fat can accelerate things further. These foods are not only quick to absorb, they're easy to eat quickly. The speed of intake compounds the speed of conversion.

Soft foods matter here as well. Anything that requires little chewing or effort often enters the system faster than expected, even if the ingredient list looks reasonable.

Protein behaves differently depending on context. When protein arrives into an already fast-moving system, it can amplify that pace. When it arrives later — into a system that's already working — it tends to settle in rather than accelerate things.

This is why food context matters more than food labels.

A food that feels destabilising on an empty stomach can feel completely neutral when it arrives later in a meal. The same bite behaves differently depending on the speed that's already been set.

Meals that begin with fast-moving foods often feel compressed. Hunger returns early. Energy spikes and drops. The body spends the rest of the day correcting.

Meals that begin more slowly can absorb these same foods without issue.

Nothing mysterious is happening.

Digestion is managing flow.

Once you start noticing which foods tend to accelerate the opening, you don't need to avoid them. You only need to decide whether they set the pace — or ride one that's already in motion.

That distinction alone changes how meals feel afterward.

Refeed Days and Keto-Leaning Examples

Refeed days exist to **restore energy without restarting instability**.

This is not a recommendation to eat a certain way, but an explanation of why different refeed styles produce different transitions.

They are not meant to feel restrictive, and they are not meant to erase the contrast created by quieter days. Their job is to feed the system while keeping signals orderly enough that digestion still finishes its work.

For some people, this happens naturally.

They eat, feel satisfied, and appetite settles without much thought. For others — especially those coming from long periods of constant eating or insulin resistance — what arrives on refeed days matters a little more.

This is where keto-leaning choices can help.

Keeping carbohydrates lower on refeed days isn't a rule. It's a way of preserving the fat-burning state that quieter days establish, while still eating enough to feel nourished and steady.

The difference shows up most clearly when refeed days are compared.

When a refeed day is treated like a feast day — heavy in refined starches or sugars — digestion often accelerates early. Insulin rises sharply. The fat-burning state ends quickly. Hunger may return sooner, and the following quieter days can feel harder to settle into.

When a refeed day leans more toward protein, fats, vegetables, and fibrous foods, energy still comes in — but at a pace the system can manage. Insulin rises enough to support eating without fully shutting down fat use. The contrast with quieter days remains intact.

This is why some people notice that Wednesday matters.

A quieter Wednesday that stays relatively low in fast-converting carbohydrates often allows the body to continue burning stored fuel through the following days. Treating Wednesday like Sunday can shorten that window.

Neither choice is wrong.

They simply lead to different outcomes.

Keto-leaning examples on refeed days often include:

- proteins that feel sustaining rather than heavy,
- vegetables that still require digestion,
- fats that slow absorption,
- simple meals that don't stack multiple fast inputs at once.

These are not prescriptions.

They're patterns that tend to **extend metabolic quiet** instead of interrupting it.

The important thing is understanding the tradeoff.

More carbohydrates bring faster replenishment — and faster exit from fat-burning.
Fewer carbohydrates preserve contrast — and often make the following quieter days easier.

Once that's clear, refeed days stop being confusing.

They become another dial you can adjust — not to optimise perfectly, but to choose how quickly the system transitions between states.

And like everything else in this book, the right setting is the one that makes eating demand less attention over time.

The Fast Meal vs Slow Meal Test

This experiment isn't about proving anything.

It's about noticing a difference that most people have felt before — without knowing why.

Choose a meal you already eat.

Don't change the foods.
Don't change the portions.
Don't improve anything.

On one occasion, eat it the way it usually happens.

Start with whatever is fastest.
Eat without pauses.
Let the meal arrive all at once.

Afterward, notice what happens.

How long before hunger returns.
Whether energy rises smoothly or drops sharply.
Whether you start thinking about food again sooner than
expected.

On another day, eat the same meal — but change the order.

Begin with something that takes time to break down. Vegetables,
soup, protein, anything textured. Give it a few minutes. Let
digestion start working before the rest arrives.

Then eat the remainder of the meal as normal.

That's the only difference.

Again, notice what happens.

Not just immediately — but over the next few hours.

Does hunger return later?
Does it feel softer?
Does the urge to "top up" fade more easily?

There's nothing to track here.

No numbers.
No targets.
No judgment.

The value of this experiment is that it removes belief from the
equation. The body gives feedback quickly when the pace
changes.

Most people find that the slow-start version holds longer — even
though the food was identical. The difference isn't the meal. It's

the sequence.

Once you've felt that contrast, you don't need to be convinced.

You've experienced how pace shapes outcome.

And that understanding carries forward into every meal without effort.

The Quiet Day Contrast

A Post-Method Self-Test

This is not a diet experiment.

You are not testing food quality, calories, discipline, or willpower.
You are not testing whether fasting "works."

You are testing **how your body behaves when digestion is repeatedly interrupted versus when it is allowed to complete.**

This appendix exists to confirm that you can now *feel* the difference described throughout the book.

What this test is measuring

This test compares **two internal states:**

- A day where digestion is **continually restarted**

- A day where digestion is **allowed to run to completion**

Nothing else is meant to change.

You are not trying to eat better on the second day.

You are not trying to eat less.
You are not trying to be disciplined.

You are observing **signal behaviour**.

How to run the contrast

Choose two ordinary days, close together.

They should be:

- similar workdays

- similar activity levels

- similar sleep

- similar stress

Do not prepare for either day.
Do not compensate.
Do not optimise food choices.

The more normal the days are, the clearer the contrast becomes.

Day One — Continuous Interruption State

On the first day, eat the way a modern, busy day naturally unfolds.

Food appears often.
Eating is opportunistic.
Drinks may contain calories or sweetness.
Snacks appear between tasks.
Eating happens in response to dips, breaks, or convenience.

Key characteristics of this day:

- Digestion is restarted before it finishes

- Insulin rarely returns to baseline

- Hunger signals overlap

- Appetite stays mentally present

- Energy feels managed rather than settled

What to notice:

- how often food enters your thoughts

- whether hunger ever fully resolves

- whether appetite feels quiet or background-active

- whether energy feels steady or continually adjusted

Do not judge this day.
This is your **baseline state**.

Day Two — Completed Digestion State

On the second day, you change **only one variable**: interruption frequency.

This is not a forced fast.
You still eat if hunger appears.

What changes is **containment**.

Eating is clear and deliberate.
Meals are distinct events.

Snacks are minimal or absent.
There is space between inputs.

Drinks on Day Two

Drinks on Day Two should be **non-sweet**.

Avoid:

- sugar

- juice

- honey

- artificially sweetened drinks

This is not a permanent rule.
It applies only to this test.

Sweet taste — even without calories — can keep appetite signalling active and maintain food attention. For this contrast, the goal is to remove **signal noise**.

Water, mineral water, plain tea, and plain coffee are appropriate.

What to notice on Day Two

Hunger may rise higher at first.

This is expected.

You are not observing intensity.
You are observing **shape**.

Notice:

- whether hunger comes in waves instead of constant background presence

- whether hunger peaks and then softens on its own

- whether food occupies less mental attention between meals

- whether energy feels calmer, not higher

Many people notice:

- fewer food thoughts

- less internal negotiation

- less need to manage energy

- a sense that the body is finishing something

A note on signal clarity

If you normally consume sweets, refined carbohydrates, or sweetened drinks between meals, appetite signals may take **a few days** to become fully clear.

This is not resistance or failure.
It reflects how hunger and insulin rhythms adapt to repeated interruption.

As interruptions stop, signals often sharpen quickly.

If the contrast feels muted on the first attempt, repeat the test after a few quieter days. Most people find the difference becomes more obvious, not harder.

The key insight this test reveals

Most people assume frequent eating keeps hunger quieter.

This test shows the opposite.

Hunger that is constantly interrupted often stays active all day. Hunger that is allowed to peak and resolve often becomes quieter overall.

Relief does not come from eating more often.
It comes from letting signals complete.

What this test is not asking you to decide

This test is not asking:

- which day you prefer

- which day is "healthier"

- whether you should eat this way every day

It is asking you to **recognise the difference**.

Once you can feel that difference clearly, the role of quiet days, fast days, and weekly rhythm stops feeling abstract.

They stop being rules.
They start being **mechanical allowances**.

Why this matters

Most modern eating never allows digestion to complete.

This test lets you feel:

- what unfinished digestion feels like

- what completed digestion feels like

Once you have felt both states consciously, you have a reference point you can return to — even when life becomes noisy.

That reference is the real outcome of this appendix.

Appendix

How to Use This Appendix

You do not need to read these papers.
You do not need to agree with every interpretation.
You do not need to reconcile them into a unified theory.

If the method described in this book produces quieter hunger, steadier energy, and less friction around food, that outcome stands on its own.

This appendix exists for readers who want to know that the observations described here are not isolated — that they sit within a broader understanding of how human appetite is regulated.

Nothing more is required.

Appendix A — Scope and Use

This book is not a medical treatment and does not replace individual medical advice.

The ideas presented here are intended for generally healthy adults exploring appetite regulation, meal pacing, and eating rhythm. If you are pregnant, managing a medical condition that affects metabolism, or recovering from an eating disorder, this approach may not be appropriate without professional guidance.

Nothing in this book requires ignoring hunger, pushing through distress, or tolerating discomfort for its own sake. Persistent or worsening symptoms are signals to pause and reassess — not challenges to overcome.

The goal throughout is stability and quiet, not endurance.

Appendix B — A Final Note on Letting the Method Fade

This appendix is here to support understanding, not to add more to manage.

If you've worked through these examples, you already have what you need.

The goal is not to remember every detail.
It's not to apply everything perfectly.
It's not to "stay on the method."

In fact, the method works best when it becomes less visible.

As meals slow and signals finish more often, eating tends to take up less space. Decisions simplify. Hunger becomes clearer. The need to intervene drops away.

That's success.

If you find yourself thinking about food less — that's the signal.
If meals hold without effort — that's the signal.
If days pass without constant negotiation — that's the signal.

There's no finish line to cross here.

There's just a point where the structure has done its job, and attention moves elsewhere.

That's when you know it's working.

Appendix C — Research Context, Not Proof

This book was written from observation first, not from literature review.

The patterns described here were noticed in lived experience long before they were mapped against academic domains. Meals that held. Hunger that softened. Weeks that behaved differently when contrast was introduced.

Only afterward did it become clear that these observations sat across well-established areas of physiology — not as a new theory, but as a particular way of arranging familiar mechanisms.

This appendix exists for readers who want to explore that context.

It is not meant to validate the method through authority, nor to argue with competing frameworks. The studies listed below do not "prove" the book. They simply show where its ideas intersect with existing research traditions.

No single paper here stands alone.
No list here is exhaustive.
None are required for the method to work.

They are included as orientation, not instruction.

Appetite Regulation & Energy Homeostasis

Much of what is experienced as hunger, craving, or loss of control emerges from central regulatory systems rather than conscious choice.

These works describe how appetite is integrated, modulated, and adjusted in response to internal signals — not willpower.

- Schwartz MW et al. — *Central nervous system control of food intake*

- Morton GJ et al. — *Neurobiology of food intake and energy balance*

- Hall KD et al. — *Energy balance and its components*

These domains inform the book's framing of hunger as a signal that can misfire under unstable conditions, rather than a simple reflection of need.

Insulin Dynamics & Postprandial Response

Insulin is often discussed in extremes — either as irrelevant or as a singular cause.

The work referenced here treats insulin more narrowly: as a signal that responds to the **rate and repetition** of incoming energy.

- Cahill GF — *Fuel metabolism in starvation*

- Jenkins DJA et al. — *Glycemic index and postprandial glucose response*

- Wolever TMS — *Carbohydrate metabolism and insulin dynamics*

These sources support the book's focus on **speed and sequence**, rather than macronutrient elimination or calorie arithmetic.

Meal Timing & Circadian Metabolism

The body does not respond to food identically at all times of day.

Circadian biology helps explain why identical meals can feel different depending on when and how often they occur.

- Panda S — *Circadian rhythms and metabolism*

- Sutton EF et al. — *Early time-restricted feeding and metabolic markers*

- Johnston JD — *Physiological responses to meal timing*

This research aligns with the book's emphasis on rhythm — not precision — and on predictability rather than optimisation.

Gastric Emptying, Food Structure & Satiety

Two meals with similar energy content can behave very differently once digestion begins.

Food structure, texture, and form influence how quickly energy enters circulation and how long satiety signals persist.

- Holt SHA et al. — *A satiety index of common foods*

- Jenkins DJA et al. — *Food form, fiber, and digestion speed*

- Cassidy A et al. — *Dietary structure and postprandial response*

These domains support the idea that **how a meal unfolds** often matters more than its ingredient list.

Stress, Signal Noise & Appetite Variability

Stress does not create hunger out of nothing, but it can amplify and distort existing signals.

The work below provides context for why appetite can feel unpredictable during periods of load, even when intake remains unchanged.

- Adam TC & Epel ES — *Stress, eating behavior, and reward pathways*
- Dallman MF et al. — *Chronic stress and energy balance*

These findings align with the book's distinction between hunger as information and hunger as noise.

A Note on What Is Not Included

This appendix deliberately avoids:

- diet-comparison trials,

- population-level correlation studies,

- advocacy-driven nutrition frameworks,

- and outcome-focused weight-loss competitions.

Not because those bodies of work are without value, but because they answer different questions.

This book is not about which diet wins.
It is about why eating systems become unstable — and how stability changes behavior downstream.

The sources listed here were chosen because they illuminate **mechanism**, not because they prescribe outcomes.

Using This Book Over Time

You do not need to remember everything in this book.

You may not need it at all once the structure settles.

Most readers return to different sections at different times — not to apply rules, but to recalibrate when eating starts to feel noisy again. A single reread of a chapter, an experiment revisited, or a reminder of pacing is often enough.

If meals are holding, hunger is arriving clearly, and food has faded into the background, the book has done its job.

There is no requirement to stay "on" anything.
There is no schedule to maintain.
There is nothing to complete.

Use this book when something feels off.
Put it down when things feel quiet.

That is how it's meant to work.

Author's Note

This book emerged from long-term observation, experimentation, and lived experience rather than from a single discipline or framework. It was written to make sense of patterns that repeated across different eating styles, schedules, and levels of effort — and to explain why some changes consistently quieted appetite while others did not.

The intent has never been to promote a particular way of eating, but to describe conditions under which eating becomes simpler.

Supplemental Note (Optional) — A Time-Limited Targeted Intervention

This section is intentionally placed at the end of the book because it introduces higher physiological load and requires a clear boundary.

This pattern is not appropriate for everyone. It should not be used by individuals who are underweight, pregnant or breastfeeding, managing an active eating disorder, recovering from disordered eating, or experiencing medical conditions where prolonged absence of intake is contraindicated. It is also not intended for those already within a healthy metabolic range who are eating calmly and maintaining stability without effort. If you have been advised by a clinician to eat regularly for medical reasons, or if periods without food reliably worsen symptoms rather than quiet them, the core pacing method described earlier is the correct stopping point. When in doubt, this application should be discussed with a qualified healthcare professional before use.

Everything required for health, metabolic stability, and long-term maintenance has already been covered. For most readers, the method as described is sufficient and complete.

What follows is not an extension of the core system. It is a **time-limited application** for a narrower group of people: those whose primary goal is **defined fat loss**, and who prefer short periods of clear structure over prolonged daily restraint.

It is optional.

It is not a lifestyle.
It is not a progression.

If this does not clearly apply to you, you can stop reading here without missing anything essential.

When Fat Loss Is the Primary Goal

Weight loss in this framework is not achieved by eating less every day.

It occurs when the body is given **longer, cleaner periods of absence**, while still preserving appetite resolution and signal clarity on eating days. That requires **fewer eating events**, not tighter control within them.

For some people, a single weekly eating pause produces steady, gradual change. For others — particularly those carrying significant weight or seeking a defined reduction phase — progress can feel slow.

This pattern exists for those situations.

It increases fat-loss pressure without introducing daily restriction, tracking, or constant negotiation.

An Author's Note

This is the structure I used during a period of significant weight loss.

Not because it was the hardest version, but because it was the cleanest.

It removed negotiation and replaced daily restraint with a small number of clear boundaries.

Once the weight was gone, I did not continue using it. I returned to the standard rhythm described earlier — because maintenance requires stability, not pressure.

That distinction matters.

A Two-Window Structure

This application uses **two discrete eating pauses** within the same week:

- a primary 48-hour absence

- a secondary 36–48-hour absence, depending on tolerance and lifestyle

Both rely on the same condition:

Absence must be complete, or the window does not function as intended.

This is not about endurance. It is about clarity of signal.

Window One — Entry and Primary Absence

The first window mirrors the standard rhythm described earlier.

Sunday functions as an entry day.

Meals are structured, fibre-forward, protein-centred, and free of added sugar or refined carbohydrates. The goal is not restriction, but reduction of volatility before absence.

Monday and Tuesday form the primary fasting window.

No food is consumed.
No liquids containing calories, fibre, or food particles are included.

This window performs the majority of the metabolic work.

Wednesday — Controlled Re-Entry

Wednesday is not a feast.

It is a buffer.

Food re-enters carefully, using the same sequencing described earlier:
acid, vegetables, protein.

Carbohydrates and heavy fats are deliberately excluded.

This is not optional.

The role of Wednesday is to stabilise appetite and settle digestion so the second window is tolerable rather than chaotic. Skipping this step usually leads to louder hunger and poorer outcomes.

Window Two — Secondary Absence

After a successful re-entry, the second absence begins.

In the standard configuration:
eating stops Wednesday evening,
Thursday and Friday form the second fasting window,
and food resumes Friday evening or Saturday morning.

Some people prefer to shift this earlier to protect social time at the end of the week. That version is harder, not easier, and should only be used when necessary.

Thursday and Friday are not "light days."
They are absence days.

Attempts to soften them with soups, broths, or "technically allowed" liquids usually re-activate digestion and undermine the window.

Saturday — Recovery

Saturday restores eating using pacing and sequence.

There is no need to restrict quantity.

The goal is to:

- restore energy gradually,

- settle hunger,

- and prevent rebound behaviour.

If Saturday becomes chaotic, the structure is too aggressive. That is feedback, not failure.

Why This Works — and Why It's Optional

Two extended absences in a single week significantly increase time spent in low-insulin, low-correction states. This increases fat-loss pressure.

It also increases systemic load.

That is why this pattern is:

- time-limited,

- deliberate,

- and explicitly optional.

Many people use it for a defined period — for example, a month — then return to the single-window rhythm once weight loss is complete.

That is expected.

Choosing the Right Structure

If your priority is:

- health,

- metabolic calm,

- long-term steadiness,

the core method is sufficient.

If your priority is:

- fat loss,

- a defined reduction phase,

- a time-limited intervention,

this pattern exists as a tool.

Neither approach reflects discipline or commitment. They serve different goals.

The only mistake is drifting between them without clarity.

When the goal changes, the structure should change with it —
deliberately, not reactively.

9 781764 523912